CANNABIS PHARMACY OIL

Cannabis Properties, Strains, Medical Usage, Thc And Cbd

By

Doreen Weed

TABLE OF CONTENTS

INTRODUCTION TO CANNABIS 9

MODERN HERBAL MEDICINE 11

    Misguided Judgments About Alternative Medicine.......... 20

CANNABIS HISTORY, PROPERTIES AND PRODUCTS 22

    Properties 26

    Cannabis Products 28

        1. Cannabis Oil 29

        2. Cannabis Beauty and Skin Care Products................. 30

        3. Cannabis Beverages 31

        4. Cannabis Chocolates...................................... 32

        5. Cannabis Gummies 33

        6. Cannabis Capsules 34

        7. Cannabis Dog Treats 34

MEDICAL CANNABIS: 36

HOW TO CHOOSE AND USE.. 36

    Instructions to Choose... 37

    Tranquilizer... 40

    Step By Step Instructions To Use 40

CANNABIS PHENOTYPE AND GENOTYPE 44

    The Earliest Cannabis Species.................................... 45

    Cannabis in the Great Indoors 46

    The Age of Hybridization 46

    The Basics: Debunking the Indica versus Sativa Binary. 48

    Genotype Versus Phenotypes..................................... 49

    Characterizing Cannabis sativa 50

CANNABIS STRAINS 51

Strains of Cannabis – Indica Versus Sativa Versus Hybrid
.... 51

Sources... 51

Consequences for The Body.............................. 52

Plant Appearance and Growth 53

DIFFERENCE BETWEEN THC AND CBD STRAINS 55

THC Dominant Marijuana Strains 55

CBD Dominant Marijuana Strains...................... 55

Adjusted CBD and THC Marijuana Strains 56

A Note On Terpenes.. 57

Most popular strains of cannabis 59

Picking the Right Cannabis Strain for You...................... 62

Conceivable Side Effects of THC Marijuana Dominant
Strains 63

GREENHOUSE CULTIVATION OF CANNABIS FOR SEEDS
USED IN PRODUCTION OF CANNABIS PHARMACY OIL
.... 65

Plan for Expansion from the Start 65

Parity Production Efficiencies.......................... 66

Building the Ideal Environment....................... 67

Picking Your Perfect Cannabis Seed for Production 71

PRODUCTION OF CANNABIS 73

PHARMACY OIL.. 73

Production and Extraction of CBD Oil............................. 75

Comparing CBD Oil Extraction Methods 76

Extra CBD Extract Processing 79

Cleansing by means of Winterization.............. 80

How CBD Isolate is Made? 80

CANNABIS PHARMACY OILS AND ITS USAGE 82

Getting THC and CBD 82

Source 82

How it Impact the body 83

The Advantages 83

Taking Internally Cannabis Oil Can: 85

The Amount to Take: 85

How Hemp Seed Oil Can Help Your Arthritis 86

The Use of High-Cannabidiol Cannabis Extracts to Treat
Epilepsy and Other Diseases 87

Cannabis Oil a Cancer Treatment Alternative to
Chemotherapy? 89

How CBD Oil Helps in Apoptosis 89

USEFULNESS OF CANNABIS OIL FOR THE AGED 95

1. Relief from discomfort 96

2. Bone Health 96

3. Mitigating Effects 96

4. Battles Glaucoma 97

5. A Sleeping Disorder and Sleep Issues 97

6. Option in contrast to Prescription Medications 98

7. Animates Appetite 98

8. Alzheimer's and Dementia 98

CANNABIS PHARMACY OIL ON PETS 99

How Is CBD Controlled to Animals? 99

How does CBD work in animals? 100

NEGATIVE IMPLICATIONS OF CANNABIS ABUSE ON GENERAL
AND ORAL HEALTH 105

Impacts on general health 106

Consequences for mental health 106

Effects on oral health 107

Cannabis use causes oral malignant growth 107

RELATED EFFECTS ON USAGE OF CANNABIS PHARMACY OIL
.... 109

Interaction with Pharmaceutical Drugs 113

Reactions of FDA-Approved Drug for Epilepsy 114

What Are the Drugs That CBD Interacts With? 115

Prodrug 116

Wellbeing Concerns 117

When Should You Avoid CBD Oil? 119

IS ALL CANNABIS OIL THE SAME? 121

Hemp Oil versus CBD Oil 122

What to Look for When You Buy CBD Oil 127

ALTERNATIVES TO CANNABIS PHARMACY OIL 129

Cannabidiol and Cancer 134

LAWS AND REGULATIONS ON MEDICINAL CANNABIS AROUND
THE WORLD 136

RECOMMENDATIONS 151

CONCLUSION 154

Cannabis is a plant that is a noteworthy wellspring of confusion for a few. While the realities show that a couple of kinds of hemp are unlawful as a result of the substance THC, which is a psychoactive molecule, not the total of the sorts of Hemp contain THC. Cannabis oil got prominence with the prosperity mindful of the world during the 1990s. For an impressive period of time people used the oil until it was removed from the market since oil is delivered utilizing the seeds of the cannabis plant. The DEA endeavored to express that the oil was illegal, anyway in HIA versus DEA it was settled that hemp-based sustenance things, including Cannabis oil were cleared from the Controlled Substances Act.

Today, Cannabis oil returns to its seat at the most noteworthy purpose of the universe of sustenance and the remedial world. It is basic to observe that there are a couple of different sorts of Cannabis oil. There is an expeller pressed grouping, which is a sustenance type thing. It is used in sustenance and embellishing specialists. Likewise, steam distilled major oil is made using the hemp seed, which is also used in the area of excellence in care and fragrance-based treatment practices. This is the expeller pressed sustenance thing we're talking about. The use of the Marijuana plant started in China about 2300 B.C. sooner or later.

According to Chinese feelings, the plant contains the solution for endlessness. The Chinese similarly used Cannabis oil to treat Malaria, menstrual issues and productivity. In the tenth century, the Indians began to use the oil to treat indigestion, and anorexia similarly to external wounds and infections, asthma, menstrual torment and anything is possible from that point. The plant fiber was used to produce textiles, sails and ropes until the start of this century. Nonetheless, taking into account the genuine concern that it is usually pleasing, various interactions will eventually make the hemp strands surface.

Cannabis oil is rich with unsaturated fats and fundamental unsaturated fats. Around 30-35% of the greatness of the hemp seeds is the oil, which is crushed out in the age of the oil. The oil contains the essential unsaturated fats OMEGA 3 and OMEGA 6 at a perfect high rate, many equivalents to chest milk. The oil in like manner contains protein, central supplements and minerals, which makes it an ideal dietary improvement. Fundamental unsaturated fats are the establishments of authentic sustenance rebuilding and repairing the body from infection. To be sure, even in the excellence care items industry, Cannabis oil drives the way. Clinical studies have shown that Cannabis oil is particularly amazing in recovering extraordinary skin issue, for instance, atopic dermatitis quite far up to devours.

Hemp oil sustains the protected structure, keeps up a strong cardiovascular system, and is amazing in helping the body fight a not unimportant once-over of conditions, for instance, cutting down "horrendous" cholesterol, raising "incredible" cholesterol, cutting down heartbeat and decreasing the threat of respiratory disappointment, similarly as being quieting. In case you are a danger sufferer and are encountering chemotherapy, using Cannabis oil is recommended all the while. It invigorates sound cell creation and decreases the damage to the body on account of treatment. The oil doesn't battle with ordinary restorative drugs and isn't a fix, yet rather is complimentary. In 1995, Deborah Gez made Moriah Herbs, and brought more than 30 years of experience to the field of home developed drug. Moriah Herbs is a pioneer in aroma-based treatment, central oils and home developed repairing.

The use of plants as medicines originates from human history and archeological evidence shows that during the Paleolithic period (around 60,000 years before) we used restorative plants. In Mesopotamia the Sumerians made mud tablets with arrangements of many restorative plants, (for example, myrrh and opium) and the Ancient Egyptians composed the Ebers Papyrus around 1500 BC, which contains data on more than 850 plant medicines, including garlic, juniper, cannabis, castor bean, aloe, and mandrake. In India the utilization of herbs to treat infirmities shapes an enormous piece of Ayurvedic prescription and obviously everybody knows about how plants and herbs are utilized widely in conventional Chinese Medicine.

The Greeks brought herbalism into the cutting-edge age and evacuated a significant part of the supernatural quality and enchantment which were available in prior writings. Hippocrates specifies 250 helpful herbs in his incredible works, and a Greek Physician named Dioscorides distributed a book called De Materia Medica which contained more than 600 restorative plants. Another Greek Galen delivered itemized abstracts on medication which included in excess of 600 plants and these were deciphered and counseled by doctors the world over for a long time. All through the Medieval time frame physical and otherworldly wellbeing kept on being upheld for the most part with plants and herbs. This treatment was typically done by priests and nuns who gave nursing administrations, with the Benedictine religious communities known for their top to bottom learning of herbals. They tended nurseries that developed the herbs which were viewed as helpful for the treatment of the different human ills. The priests additionally invested a lot of their energy deciphering old style chips away at herbalism into Latin and creating "Herbals" to be utilized by doctors.

The fifteenth, sixteenth, and seventeenth hundreds of years were the extraordinary period of herbals, huge numbers of them accessible without precedent for English and different dialects instead of Latin or Greek. Close by the customary acts of Herbalism there were many learned men of science and prescription who accepted sickness was brought about by "terrible humor" in the body that must be driven out and discharged. The popular American specialist Benjamin Rush, Treasurer of the Mint, and endorser of the Declaration of Independence, wrote numerous restorative course books, in which he prescribed splashing patients with cold water in the winter, spinning patients from ropes suspended from the roof for a considerable length of time, just as beating, starving and obnoxiously mishandling patients. He additionally poured corrosive on their backs and cut them with blades enabling the injuries to be kept open for a considerable length of time or years, to encourage "perpetual release of awful humor from the cerebrum".

When King Charles II woke up feeling sick his Royal Barber took 16 ounces of blood, and his primary care physicians depleted a further eight ounces. He was made to swallow antimony, a poisonous metal, and given a progression of bowel purges. At the point when his sickness proceeded with Charles' head was shaved and rankling operators were applied to his scalp, to drive the awful humor descending. Pigeon droppings were applied to the bottoms of Charles' feet, and more blood was drawn. He was given white sugar treats, to float his spirits, and nudged with a super-hot poker. He was then given 40 drops of seepage from "the skull of a man that was rarely covered" what its identity was, guaranteed, had kicked the bucket a roughest passing. At long last, squashed stones from the inner parts of a goat from East India were constrained down his throat. Charles II kicked the bucket on February 6, 1685.

In the eighteenth century anyway, doctors tried to turn out to be progressively logical and there were numerous self-prepared stylist specialists, pharmacists, maternity specialists, medicate vendors, and pretenders who were rehearsing medicine right now. In any case, the town Wise Women could in any case be depended on to supply customary herbs or blends to treat minor sicknesses and this training kept on being prevalent with the common laborers who couldn't bear to pay doctor's expenses. Samuel Thomson was a self-instructed ranch kid who took in herbalism from a nearby shrewd lady and composed a book enumerating these techniques, this book was well known to the point that pretty much every home had a duplicate (together with a book of scriptures) and it was even taken on wagon-prepares and conveyed over the USA.

The American Medical Association came into control towards the finish of the nineteenth Century and the logical insurgency lessened the prevalence of herbalism and presented a time of perilous medical practices presented by the recently framed pharmaceutical industry. During this period Paracelsus presented the utilization of dynamic synthetic medications (like arsenic, copper sulfate, iron, mercury, and sulfur). On the off chance that you were a focus on nineteenth century mother you could now buy for your kids a progression of "alleviating syrups," tablets and powders which in reality contained hazardous opiates, for example, morphine sulfate, chloroform, morphine hydrochloride, codeine, heroin, powdered opium, and cannabis indica," and some of the time a few of them in mix. Heroin was likewise usually used to treat hacks!

Mercury was utilized much of the time to treat numerous normal infirmities. Mercury, as we presently know, is dangerous to the body and side effects of mercury harming incorporate chest agonies, heart and lung issues, hacking, tremors, savage muscle fits, insane responses, incoherence, pipedreams, and even self-destructive inclinations! Numerous post-mortem examinations uncovered "Silver Liver Syndrome" to be the reason for death during this period. Present day medicine then "advanced" considerably more to incorporate radical medications like phlebotomy, leeches, and exploratory techniques like lobotomies and electric stun medicines. Trepanation, boring openings in the head, was another well-known treatment and was most ordinarily utilized for seizures and headaches!

"Diet pills" were presented during the 1920s and '30s which were in truth containers loaded up with got dried out tapeworms or tapeworm eggs. In the 1950s and 1960s new pills were being sold that vowed to soften away those pounds and inches yet these could cause fevers, heart inconveniences, visual deficiency, demise and birth abandons. Those eating routine pills were massively addictive and in truth contained unadulterated amphetamines. Since the beginning of current medicine, the pharmaceutical business has fortunately advanced and controls are set up to guarantee pharmaceutical medications and medicines are ok for us to utilize. Without a doubt physician recommended medications can spare and change lives. I entirely support and embrace that you keep on utilizing any professionally prescribed medicine which you might be at present taking and ought not to quit ingesting any recommended medications without counseling your primary care physician first.

In any case, it is irrefutable that close by the advantages which physicians recommended medications can offer they can likewise accompany unwelcome symptoms. Record quantities of patients are enduring or kicking the bucket because of physician endorsed medication symptoms. Some generally recorded and demonstrated symptoms from physician recommended medications extend from cerebral pains, tiredness, skin responses, stoppage, looseness of the bowels, gastrointestinal issues, stomach hurts, water gauge addition, joint and muscle torment and diminished authority over real works, loss of taste, amnesia, locate misfortune, mental trips, sickness and heaving causing lack of hydration, inner draining and esophageal break, through to unfavorably susceptible responses that can deliver an anaphylactic reaction in patients, serious torment, aggregate or incomplete loss of motion, strokes, muscle agony and loss of muscle co-appointment, blood clusters, coronary episodes, congestive cardiovascular breakdown, deep rooted heart harm and cardiomyopathy and incredibly even malignant growth. Physician endorsed medications have additionally been connected to misery and self-destructive contemplations.

Well that is a significant not insignificant rundown of realized reactions from taking physician endorsed medications, and this is in no way, shape or form a total list! You will locate a comparable rundown of perilous known symptoms from the synthetic substances found in our regular family unit items - the normal American home contains more than 63 dangerous items including antiperspirants and antiperspirants, scents, toilet bowl cleaners, over-the-counter meds, pills, creams, gels and so on., healthy skin items, and "deodorizers". These items contain many synthetic mixes that are conceivably perilous.

Numerous ordinary items like cleansers and shampoos, cleaning up fluid or air pocket shower, even toothpaste - in certainty anything which froths, as often as possible contains a fixing known as Sodium Lauryl Ether Sulfate which can cause extreme skin and eye aggravation, loose bowels, sensory system melancholy, worked breathing and in uncommon cases demise. Parabens are another basic fixing we can discover in shampoos, business creams, shaving gels, individual ointments, topical/parenteral pharmaceuticals, shower tanning arrangement, cosmetics, and toothpaste and are likewise typical nourishment added substance. Parabens have been appeared to cause skin bothering and contact dermatitis and rosacea in people with paraben hypersensitivities and all the more worryingly they can impersonate the female hormone estrogen and have been found in bosom malignancy tumors and connected with the early beginning of pubescence in young ladies.

Another lethal fixing found in numerous family unit cleaners is Butoxyethanol which whenever assimilated through the skin can harm your blood, liver and kidneys and another concoction which is known to cause kidney harm is Perchloroethylene which is usually found in cover cleaners. A fixing found in window cleaning arrangements is Diethylene Glycol is known to discourage the sensory system and most toilet cleaners contain a large group of unsafe synthetic compounds and acids which could cause visual impairment in a flash, and are harmful to the respiratory and circulatory frameworks. Maybe one of the most stunning contaminations in our house is the regularly utilized deodorizers which contain substances called phthalates (articulated Thalates), which are incredibly perilous and known to cause hormonal variations from the norm, conceptive issues and even birth absconds. Worryingly the names on all these regular ordinary family items are frequently deceptive and mistaking for bundling proposing items are "all common", and so forth when in truth they contain various poisons.

Obviously, there is presently a developing pattern to utilize increasingly normal items in our homes and on our bodies. Numerous individuals are deliberately detoxing their homes and ways of life by coming back to customary strategies and by and by making our own cleaning items, excellence items, and individual care items like toothpaste, cleanser, face cream just as utilizing unadulterated normal items like plants and herbs by and by to battle minor illnesses and advance great health.

Presently, in these modern occasions it would be hard for us to turn the clock back as we may wish and recapture the learning once went from age to age about how to utilize Mother Nature's plants and herbs to keep up our great health and stay away from the requirement for conceivably lethal synthetic concoctions in our ordinary family unit and excellence items and physician recommended drugs. Quite a bit of that information has been lost and a significant number of those fixings and strategies would not be useful for us to utilize any more.

So, What Decisions Do We Have on The Off Chance That We Need to Bring Our Families Up in An Increasingly Common Manner?

Numerous individuals have found humankind's most productive technique for rehearsing herbalism - they utilize 100% unadulterated basic oils, which contain the "soul of the plants". Basic oils are the exceptionally focused, fragrant embodiments of trees, bushes, herbs, grasses, gums and blooms. Restorative evaluation oils can be utilized fragrantly either legitimately breathed in or diffused, topically (applied to the skin), or now and again taken inside (ingested). The oils all have their own novel dynamic properties and by and large, every basic oil contains more than 100 constituents with all the more being found each day. 1 drop of unadulterated fundamental oil contains 40 million trillion particles that influence the body at the cell level. Every day, an ever-increasing number of people are changing to a cleaner way of life with fewer poisons in their homes and, like our precursors, we are actually adapting how to use the restorative properties of herbs and plants. We make our own cleaning items utilizing economical basic fixings in mix with basic oils, we make our very own self consideration items, for example, cleansers, shower salts, toothpaste, mouthwash, cleanser, child wipes, creams, and in reality each item you presently use can be imitated in a protected, common structure utilizing fundamental oils related to items like Epsom salts, olive oil, coconut oil, dark colored sugar, ocean salt, vinegar, refined water, and so on.

Right now, there is an oily upset occurring, each day an ever-increasing number of homes choose to come back to progressively customary attempted and tried strategies for homemaking and health the board. With the monstrous development that fundamental oils are encountering as we come back to utilizing more straightforward and progressively normal items in our home, there has been an ascent in modest "off the rack" impersonation basic oils which are not Therapeutic Grade oils, and are just appropriate to be utilized for their scent. A fundamental oil can legitimately be marked "unadulterated" regardless of whether it contains as meager as 5% of the genuine oil (that is just 5% of the dynamic elements of the oil). The rest of the jug is regularly loaded up with modest engineered filler synthetic compounds which have been delivered for their "scent" characteristics as it were. These oils regularly contain hurtful synthetic concoctions and potential poisons. Stay away from items named "scent" or "Parfum" as these are second rate aroma grade basic oils and may contain possibly hurtful sulfates or phthalates.

Basic Oils make them flabbergast properties which advance great health and bolster the body's common protections, they bolster the safe framework, are state of mind hoisting, fragrant, unwinding, renewing, oxygenating, purging, they help cell recovery, are high in cancer prevention agents, support stamina and vitality, improve mental lucidity, help oversee uneasiness and dissatisfaction, and advance generally speaking prosperity, essentialness, and life span!

So to summarize humankind has been using the intensity of Mother Nature's plants and herbs to advance great health and prosperity for more than 60,000 years. In the last barely any hundred years this information has gotten to some degree lost to numerous individuals as we have experienced a time of logical revelations, and medical leaps forward and these customary homes grew plans and techniques have gotten to some degree outdated. Nonetheless, there is a renaissance occurring and consistently an ever-increasing number of individuals are searching out an elective decision. The prevalence of conventional home grew plans and healthy home-made cures are developing each day. Fundamental oils are the most productive, compelling and minimal effort way that enables us to pick a progressively regular and customary way of life for our families. There is an oily transformation occurring right now as we each try to get back in agreement with Mother Nature.

MISGUIDED JUDGMENTS ABOUT ALTERNATIVE MEDICINE

Medical marijuana or MMJ has been utilized throughout recent decades to help individuals beset with genuine medical conditions that incorporate, yet are not restricted to glaucoma, malignancy, epilepsy, AIDS, and MS (Multiple Sclerosis). As one of the best specialists that assist individuals with adapting to incessant agony, medical marijuana offers patients help from extraordinary distress by easing their side effects. Understanding the science behind the adequacy of marijuana is significant so as to scatter these fantasies and settle on a very much educated decision about what it really offers. When managed under the supervision of a certified and able specialist or medical expert, medical marijuana lessens the torment and queasiness that different health issues cause. Scores of individuals accept that medical marijuana is very addictive and it builds the reliance on the medication.

Research shows that there is no proof to help this conviction in light of the fact that to begin with, medical cannabis doesn't have any synthetic concoctions that may trigger habit in individuals who use it as a piece of their treatment procedure. At that point there are different confusions that MMJ may likewise prompt the utilization of hard drugs, for example, cocaine and like the previous, this is additionally only a misinterpretation. While medical marijuana can be smoked, this isn't the main way that it tends to be utilized. Directly from doctor prescribed drugs and pills that contain manufactured types of medical marijuana to other substitute treatment strategies, cannabinoids, for example, THC can be conveyed to the body without smoking MMJ. The blooms and leaves can be absorbed a blend of liquor to remove the cannabinoids in marijuana. This mixture can either be added to beverages and nourishment or consumed through skin patches and in this structure; it takes MMJ as meager as a half hour to create the ideal impact. The dynamic parts can likewise be moved into cooking oil and spread by stewing the plant in them for a few hours. This is typically used to heat treats and brownies or make different sorts of nourishment that a patient may discover tantalizing.

Thought there are tests that show that Medical cannabis can cause momentary memory misfortune in certain patients who are experiencing treatment, actually the impact is just impermanent. Medical marijuana neither decreases their knowledge nor does it influence their long-haul memory. Despite the fact that medical cannabis is an all-common substance that is gotten from plants, the misguided judgments about it are very dubious and ridiculous.

CANNABIS HISTORY, PROPERTIES AND PRODUCTS

For many years, cannabis has been associated with humanity. Cannabis has characteristics that are psychoactive and remedial. In nature, the cannabis plant can grow up to five meters in height. It blooms in late harvest time between the fag end of the mid-year season. Some of the Chinese records written in 2800 BC were the most reliable reference to cannabis. In many Asian nations, cannabis is a wild plant. Cannabis is broadly esteemed to have begun in India. Numerous indigenous networks over the world have been utilizing cannabis for a few purposes like strict, recreational, and medical. Numerous doctors recommend meds having cannabis to patients experiencing such sicknesses as glaucoma, different sclerosis, HIV, and malignant growth, other than a few others. Cannabis in like manner gives the vim to the heart and the results have been exhibited to be a lot of equivalent to an individual rehearsing reliably in the diversion focus!

Nowadays, cannabis is perceived as a drug. Cannabis is precluded in various countries. Normally, cannabis customers prevented from securing the medicine have been viewed as commanding in nature. Toward the day's end, cannabis is addictive rationally. The effect is extremely similar to steroids that are anabolic in nature. What's more, addicts of a couple of hard medications have been viewed as the wellsprings of major sociological or health issues. However, an assessment has exhibited that cannabis customers are less disposed to make such aggravations. More than 400 manufactured mixes set up cannabis. Cannabis has been used by various indigenous people because of its psychoactive effects. The fundamental psychoactive segment in cannabis is 'THC' or tetrahydrocannabinol.

A lot of cannabis brown haze can antagonistically influence the circulatory strain process and an individual can even black out because of this impact. Individuals having a history of such health issues like dissemination and heart issue, other than schizophrenia should absolutely evade cannabis. Such individuals can have inconveniences regardless of whether they become uninvolved smokers. Routine cannabis smokers experience the evil impacts of lung threat, emphysema, and bronchitis. Thusly, the best way to deal with go without being a cannabis aficionado is to express 'NO!' to the medicine the main go through ever. There is reliably the threat of a standard cannabis customer taking to progressively destructive psychoactive medications like cocaine and heroin.

The cannabis plant is commonly referred to as hemp, marijuana or cannabis indica. Cannabis is called cannabis, tobacco, opium, pot, herb, smoke, vapor, hemp, marijuana, or ganja, unlike the different names.

Many young people around the globe have been seen stuck in marijuana, regardless of the prohibitions.

As cancer-causing agents (specialists that induce malignant growth), marijuana has more tar than tobacco.

The most grounded and focused type of cannabis oil is fabricated from the cannabis sap. The sap is broken down, separated lastly vanished. In the UK, this oil is separated by cocaine and heroin closely and is a prescription under the course of action of Class A. As squares, cannabis tar is removed from the buds of cannabis. When they are prepared for use, these cannabis squares are then warmed up and disintegrated. The shade of the cannabis sap can fluctuate from green to dim dark colored. This structure is prominently called 'hash', 'soapbar' or 'dark'. The home-grown type of cannabis is known as skunk, weed or just 'grass'. It is set up from the dried or powdered buds of the cannabis plant.

Researches on cannabis have hurled fascinating information. Take for example the discovering around 46 percent of individuals in the age bunch from 14 to 30 have been snared to cannabis regardless of whether incidentally. Moreover, 50% of these people have come back to the plant. At this point web surfing in the United States, marijuana smoking was seen as increasingly common. While in the UK, marijuana has been found to have as much as 78 percent of people kept for medicine-related offenses.

Cannabis is presently the most broadly utilized and dubious medication on the planet. While a few people shout out for stricter marijuana laws and stiffer punishments for clients and sellers, others censure lawful frameworks which rebuff peaceful "pot smokers." United States residents everything being equal and social statuses expend it, yet American government officials looking for re-appointment are hesitant to advocate its legitimateness. Generally speaking, a superior comprehension of the history, uses, and risks of marijuana can assist social orders with creating progressively productive and vote based arrangements for its guidelines.

In the same way as other personality modifying drugs, marijuana has been utilized worldwide for a large number of years. Antiquated Chinese writings portray its utilization in both recreational and medical settings.

Archeological proof proposes that the cannabis plant previously spread from Asia to Africa, and was considered developing to be Europe as right on time as the 6th century, A.D. Over a thousand years after the fact, pilgrim Americans developed hemp as a money crop for its handiness in materials.

Somewhere in the range of 1850 and 1942, American specialists routinely endorsed marijuana for help with discomfort, stomach issues, and joint pain. Cannabis was likewise utilized recreationally - and legitimately - during the majority of this time. It was not until 1935 and the death of the Uniform State Narcotic Drug Act that most states started to carefully direct the medication.

All through the 1950s and 60s, marijuana was seen fundamentally as an insubordinate, countercultural, or "radical" tranquilize." However, despite everything it didn't convey the taboos or hardened legitimate punishments that exist today. The 1970 Controlled Substances Act added to the present the norm by making marijuana a Schedule I medicate - in a similar class as heroin, cocaine, and different opiates. As a feature of the Reagan organization's War on Drugs, obligatory condemning laws went during the 1980s which still require sentences of a quarter century or more for thrice-indicted marijuana guilty parties.

These authoritative choices stay questionable right up 'til the present time, and change supporters contend that marijuana isn't about so risky or propensity framing as to require such severe legitimate punishments. They additionally much of the time push for the decriminalization of marijuana, particularly for medical use. Gatherings of these promoters are enormous and assorted, and incorporate such associations as the Coalition for Rescheduling Cannabis, Law Enforcement

Against Prohibition, and Students for Sensible Drug Policy.

Notwithstanding varying suppositions on the legitimateness and social agreeableness of marijuana, the vast majority can concur that the quantity of individuals captured for peaceful marijuana wrongdoings has become a significant issue. US correctional facilities are loaded up with a huge number of these convicts, and Congress burns through billions of citizen dollars keeping them bolted up. Besides, these guilty parties are regularly put in indistinguishable offices from killers, vicious street pharmacists, and different risky lawbreakers. They face long, life-expending sentences, and even marijuana clients who need assistance with dependence seldom approach appropriate treatment programs. Increasingly more marijuana clients wind up in the slammer, however the medication issue in America isn't improving.

Fortunately, help is accessible for the individuals who need it. On the off chance that you are battling with marijuana or other addictive substances, utilize the connections underneath for a classified conference. We are remaining by day and night to kick you off making a course for recuperation.

PROPERTIES

Marijuana contains the substance THC which is known by most of individuals yet expected without a compound hint, to be dangerous or addictive. THC, short for some long geeky name you'll easily forget at any rate, has been managed in different sub-atomic structures to malignancy, HIV and various sclerosis sufferers for a considerable length of time with apparent achievement.

Tetrahydrocannabinol (THC) is the dynamic substance in cannabis and is one of the most established psychedelic drugs known. There is proof that cannabis concentrates were utilized by the Chinese as a natural cure since the main century AD. Cannabis originates from the blooming tops and leaves of the hemp plant, Cannabis sativa (appeared in the image on the right). For a considerable length of time this plant has been generally developed far and wide for its filaments, and in reality, the word canvas, which is a material produced using woven hemp strands, takes its name from cannabis. Be that as it may, cannabis is all the more usually known as the wellspring of the marijuana tranquilizes, despite the fact that the word marijuana applies both to the entire plant, and to the sap from it (in spite of the fact that this is now and then likewise called hashish).

Cannabis contains around 60 diverse psychoactive synthetic concoctions called cannabinoids, of which the most significant one is tetrahydrocannabinol (THC). The method of activity of THC is as yet not appropriately comprehended, despite the fact that it is realized that of the two stereoisomers (identical representations), the structure (the left-gave type of the particle) is 10-15 times more intense than the (+)- structure.

The cannabinoids have a place with a class of synthetic substances called terpenoids, which means terpene-like. These mixes happen as fundamental oils inside numerous plants and some are associated with the development of nutrients, steroids, colors and scents. The fragrance business depends on mixes, for example, these, and they additionally discover an assortment of employments in the nourishment and pharmaceutical industry as flavor

27

and scent improvers. Terpenes can be direct, (for example, geraniol or citronella) or cyclic as in THC. Instances of some other straightforward cyclic terpenes are demonstrated as follows.

CANNABIS PRODUCTS

As cannabis turns out to be increasingly lawful, the industry encompassing it keeps on growing. Government officials presently crusade on a foundation of all out weed authorization since it's that famous a position, and it appears to be each other week there's a neighborhood news anecdote about a mother who turned into a mogul preparing and selling edibles. Since it has arrived at suburbia, organizations need to extend advertising endeavors.

That is in reality entirely troublesome. Noticeable web indexes like Google aren't especially enthused about letting individuals promoting marijuana products on their site, regardless of whether the express it's created in is lawful. Makers have been compelled to discover different intends to sell their products.

Regardless of these barricades, the blast in cannabis fame has implied a blast in cannabis products this decade. Since THC and CBD can enter the body from numerous points of view - smoking, vaping, ingesting, through skin - the quantity of products that can be made with it are, if not perpetual, absolutely abundant. Certain products, however, appear to be progressively noticeable, or possibly on the ascent, then others.

It ought to be noticed that this e-book isn't a support of any of the products that will be referenced. Cannabis is as yet illicit at the government level, and because of its characterization as a Schedule 1 medication the measure of research that can be led on it is constrained. This is basically an affirmation of prevalent kinds of products in states where cannabis is lawful in some structure:

1. CANNABIS OIL

This is truly a really wide classification in its own right. There are weed products we'll get the opportunity to further down that contain cannabidiol (CBD) oil to give you the ideal impacts. Be that as it may, cannabis oil can be taken without anyone else in various structures. That flexibility has made it effectively the most looked for after cannabis product for individuals searching for lawful use. CBD oils have exceedingly low hints of THC, so they won't give you the high that you'd typically partner with marijuana. That way one can possibly get the ideal impacts - help with discomfort, uneasiness alleviation, sickness help, and so forth - without psychoactive responses.

Epilepsy is the condition that appears to get the most steady help for utilization of cannabis oil, even governmentally; the U.S. Nourishment and Drug Administration (FDA) as of late got a consistent vote by their government warning council to suggest endorsement of a pharmaceutical CBD oil known as Epidiolex, which can be utilized to treat certain uncommon types of epilepsy. Be that as it may, CBD oil has additionally demonstrated itself to be helpful with respect to relief from discomfort, malignant growth treatment, nervousness, misery, and rest issues, among different conditions.

CBD oil, as its own usable element, can come in a few structures, and the bigger organizations that produce and sell them will offer an assortment of choices to browse. E-fluid for a vape pen is the most widely recognized structure, yet another is tinctures. CBD tinctures are drops of concentrated CBD extricate that are dropped under your tongue and assimilate in the mouth. There are cases as well, which can be taken with water like your normal pill.

Obviously, on the off chance that somebody who needs legitimate cannabis oil likewise doesn't need a broker, they're allowed to truly simply put CBD oil on their tongue and swallow it. CBD hemp oil is legitimately sold at certain dispensaries.

2. CANNABIS BEAUTY AND SKIN CARE PRODUCTS

As CBD utilize turned out to be increasingly across the board and cannabis turned out to be additionally sanctioned in more expresses, certain organizations and business visionaries had thoughts of showcasing these products to individuals who aren't regularly promoted weed: rural ladies. Because of this, the industry of CBD beauty products develops exponentially consistently - however it's not simply rural ladies who use them. CBD, notwithstanding the advantages referenced before, is additionally said to have mitigating properties due to cannabinoid receptors in skin. A few researchers state it might have the option to help battle skin break out, and beauty/skincare products with cannabinoids are publicized as having the option to help with relief from discomfort, hydration, or even only a euphoric loosened up feeling.

How standard are these products turning out to be? Products containing CBD are currently being sold on Sephora's site. The blend of impacts these products indicate to offer are horrendously enticing, all things considered. Cannabis demulcents ointments offer the capability of muscle relief from discomfort, while moisturizers and rubs offer the charm of more clear skin. Shower bombs and shower salts may bring some truly necessary help and unwinding in the tub. The weed topicals market is genuine, and continually extending; you would now be able to purchase marijuana body wash, lip gleam, and mascara as well. The sort of cannabinoids your beauty products have help decide the impacts. A large number of these products center around CBD and the health benefits it gives. Be that as it may, some additionally have more THC, accessible in dispensaries.

3. CANNABIS BEVERAGES

Cannabis beverages haven't arrived at the standard statures of the beauty products, yet they're getting more presentation, as prove by an ongoing article about CBD mixed drinks in Goop. Mixed drinks implanted with cannabis are still in their early stages, consigned for the most part to a couple of bars in Los Angeles, however should recreational marijuana use keep on getting sanctioned in more expresses, it's a pattern that could grow rapidly. Beverages implanted with marijuana have been consigned to states where the medication is either completely legitimized or decriminalized, acting nearly as test markets for future states. In Colorado, where recreational marijuana is legitimate, a few dispensaries - like Medicine Man, which has various areas - sell cannabis cola and fruit juice. What's more, numerous coffeehouses in New York sell cannabis-implanted espressos, for quieting down any individual who gets a bad case of nerves from a solid cup.

In any case, the one beverage that is regularly given CBD tests, it's lager. This is on the grounds that notwithstanding all the previously mentioned impacts of cannabinoids, the terpenes in cannabis offer various smells and tastes. There have been a few detours en route, especially because of government decisions around what is and isn't a Schedule 1 medication. There have been workarounds however, particularly for brewers and bottling works that stay in states with lawful weed. Keith Villa, maker of Blue Moon, is dealing with cannabis-injected non-fermented lagers in Colorado, while distilleries like Coalition Brewing have CBD lager accessible at select areas in both Oregon and Washington.

4. CANNABIS CHOCOLATES

Edibles are an especially well-known approach to get high, as they have more strength than different techniques. It likewise allows you to nibble while taking your now legitimate medicine, which is an or more. The most notable edibles are genuinely standard - the weed brownie, the pot treat, marijuana gummies (which have once in a while raised organizations to run into lawful ruckus because of concerns children may unintentionally take them).

As it gets lawful and organizations need to showcase cannabis treats, however, it is chocolates that have become something of a pattern. Chocolates can be showcased to those keen on attempting lawful weed yet who need an increasingly "refined" technique than smoking a joint. It additionally enables organizations to endeavor a more advanced advertising effort than you could do with, say, a sticky bear. Two of the more noticeable producers of marijuana chocolates, Kiva and Défoncé, each utilization a Godiva- esque plan to their wrappers. Presently you can feel extravagant eating a chocolate bar intended to get you high!

These chocolates are sold in restricted style, typically, as they contain THC. Défoncé is just sold and conveyed in California. In any case, should these advertising endeavors stay fruitful, if legitimate marijuana spreads to extra states it won't just be CA dispensaries that stocks them.

5. CANNABIS GUMMIES

Need desserts however not chocolate? Not to stress. Gummies, especially CBD-explicit gummies, have gotten one of the most prevalent products in the wake of legitimate marijuana. In spite of the fact that still in an unregulated area, which means it's difficult to decide with any genuine precision the amount CBD is truly in them, CBD gummies are presently productive enough that it's normal to see CBD sticky worms at a neighborhood service station.

Subsequently, on the off chance that you live in a state with medical marijuana and have a medical marijuana card (or live in a state with lawful recreational marijuana and are of lawful age), your nearby dispensary is sure to have sticky bears, worms and more to look over, regardless of whether with just CBD or with THC too. Organizations like Green Roads and Diamond CBD offer a gathering of CBD gummies for those where weed is lawful. Gummies are effectively one of the most pervasive choices accessible to those searching for a treat.

6. CANNABIS CAPSULES

Not as sweet as the chocolates and gummies or as reviving as a lager, capsules are a possibility for the individuals who simply need something to take care of business. Capsules are increasingly famous for the individuals who aren't searching for a nibble with their weed, deciding to rather take it like medicine - which, to numerous individuals in this nation, is the thing that it is. Capsules are frequently most mainstream for CBD use. The previously mentioned Medicine Man in Colorado, for instance, sells both CBD capsules and cannabinol (CBN) capsules. Resembling some other case pills, it's as straightforward as anyone might imagine.

7. CANNABIS DOG TREATS

Offering cannabis to your pets? Is that sheltered? Well don't give your dog a pot treats with human partitions, and be careful about anything with high THC content, however there are a few organizations that have played with making hemp and CBD products explicitly for pets. Numerous accounts of pets being effectively treated by marijuana are recounted, as getting endorsement for government research into the subject has demonstrated exceedingly troublesome and vets aren't lawfully permitted to recommend it. In any case, numerous researchers stay resolved to consider the impacts medical marijuana can have on pets, and some nearby legislators in states like California have acquainted bills with attempt and authorize endorsing cannabis for them.

More inside and out examinations would enable us to decide exactly how evident a significant number of the cases - that CBD can help pet proprietors treat malignant growth, epilepsy, osteoporosis, joint agony, and uneasiness - really are. All things considered, hemp and cannabidiol haven't demonstrated themselves to have any exceptional hazard to dogs, as long as you stay mindful; only one out of every odd organization that claims their CBD products have negligible THC is coming clean. An excessive amount of THC isn't useful for dogs. Should you have just chosen to attempt CBD for your puppy's infirmity, there are choices. Canna-pet offer hemp dog treats in a few flavors just as tinctures, which are another prevalent technique for pets as some can be exacting about treats and capsules. Dispensaries in Colorado may likewise sell treats for your dog.

Be that as it may, as referenced, be progressively cautious about cannabis products for your dog. The absence of government guideline or sufficient investigations implies there's no genuine solid assurance of what amount is a lot for dogs. Cannabis products made for pets are made carefully for down to earth purposes; don't get them high.

MEDICAL CANNABIS:

HOW TO CHOOSE AND USE

From little data to an over-burden of data on the web, it is anything but difficult to envision that a great many people living with torment, their relatives, and parental figures will be overpowered about whether cannabis is a reasonable help with discomfort alternative. Most importantly, it is critical to have a genuine discourse and settle on an educated choice, in organization with your healthcare supplier. People may have diverse medical conditions that coincide with a specific agony issue, and that may influence the decision and the conveyance technique for cannabis. All included ought to not just comprehend the various sorts (strains) of medical grade cannabis that exists, yet in addition the conveyance frameworks accessible.

Also, you have to know the run of the mill impacts of medical marijuana just as reactions that could happen. For instance, somebody with past mind damage posed me a keen inquiry, "Will cannabis fry my cerebrum?" Another individual living with asthma, communicated worries about cannabis impact on the lung whenever he breathed in through vaping. Concerns like these will affect your choice – how to choose, how to use, or regardless of whether to use. How about we talk about these issues. As a matter of first importance, there is no single, clear answer at the present time. As expressed in a past blog, Pot for Pain Relief? What the Research Gurus Say..., research discoveries are constrained, however encouraging. Getting your work done is basic.

As indicated by Marijuanadoctors.com, there are a great many strains of cannabis that exist. Most fall into three classes: indica, sativa and half breed. There are others, for example, cannabis ruderalis and modern hemp; which are not very much considered.

Indica: All the more steadying, arrives in an assortment of flavors and contains significant levels of pitch. Can come in unadulterated and mixed structures. Indica strains are developed in harsher atmospheres like the center east, Northern Africa, and Nepal. Normally recommended for the accompanying conditions:

- Help with discomfort
- Uneasiness and Stress Disorders
- Seizure Disorders
- Muscle Spasms

Sativa: All the more animating and invigorating, it may manufacture innovativeness. It furthermore comes in combination of fruity-sweet to characteristic flavors. Sativa is created in the Far East, South America and Mexico. Used, anyway not by and large prescribed, for the going with conditions:

- Distress
- Improved focus and ingenuity
- Perspective Elevation
- A resting issue

Note: Pure sativa can start sporadic heartbeats and doubt.

Half and half: regularly a mix of indica and sativa; strains are mixed for positive properties and favored characteristics. Makers (similarly called reproducers) are resolved in making a collection to address the perfect effects both by recreational and medical purchasers.

Cross breed: Ordinarily a blend of indica and sativa; strains are blended for positive properties and favored attributes. Cultivators (additionally called raisers) are tenacious in making an assortment to address the ideal impacts both by recreational and medical purchasers. Hence, most medical cannabis is cross breed, which means crossovers are normally a blend of seeds from various nations worldwide where marijuana can effectively develop. Cross breed can be used for:

- Hoisting Mood
- Invigorating Activities and Productivity
- Decline social nervousness
- Improve inspiration
- Overcome social nervousness
- Persuade your psyche
- Decline weakness
- Help with discomfort
- Lift sorrow
- Improve hunger
- Decline nausea and improve assimilation

Mixture: Commonly a blend of indica and sativa; strains are blended for positive properties and favored qualities. Cultivators (likewise called reproducers) are determined in making an assortment to address the ideal impacts both by recreational and medical customers.

In this way, most medical cannabis is half and half, which means crossovers are ordinarily a mix of seeds from various nations worldwide where marijuana can effectively develop. Half breeds can be used for:

- Lifting Mood
- Stimulating Activities and Productivity
- Diminishing social nervousness
- Improve inspiration
- Vanquish social nervousness
- Propel your psyche
- Diminishing weakness
- Relief from discomfort
- Lift melancholy
- Improve craving
- Reduction nausea and improve processing

Nod of seeds from different countries worldwide where marijuana can viably create. Half breeds can be used for:

- Raising Mood
- Stimulating Activities and Productivity
- Reducing social pressure
- Improve motivation
- Beat social pressure
- Motivate your mind
- Reduction exhaustion
- Help with inconvenience
- Lift misery
- Improve hunger
- Reduction nausea and improve handling

Strains can be used in mix, for example, with misery or exhaustion. Sativa could be suggested for daytime use. For sleep deprivation and agony, Indica may be recommended to be used around evening time. These strains regularly have one of kind names, for example,

Lemon Haze (Sativa): Happy, euphoric and elevating; assists with tension, torment, absence of craving

Jack Herer (Sativa): Cerebral, vigorous and innovative; assists with despondency, weariness, nausea

Blue Dream (Hybrid): Relaxed, tired, torment alleviating and social; assists with cerebral pains, aggravation, muscle fits

Blue God (Indica): Pain alleviation, expanded craving and a casual state; assists with sleep deprivation, stress, torment.

Medical quality stains ought to contain more CBD (cannabidiol), which has remedial impacts, than THC (tetrahydocannibidiol); THC has psychoactive properties which causes the "high" favored by recreational users.

STEP BY STEP INSTRUCTIONS TO USE

Smoking: Smoking is the most outstanding conveyance framework, where dried leaves are either folded into little cigarettes (doobie, joint, reefer), or put in a pipe or bong (water pipe), which is lit and smoke is breathed in.

Advantages: Smoking gives quick acting alleviation from torment, nausea or different side effects, the guideline of dosing is simple, lower cost and little requirement for leaf preparing in this way progressively unadulterated.

Disadvantages: Smoking isn't the best choice on the off chance that you have asthma, visit respiratory sicknesses, incessant bronchitis, COPD or lung malignant growth. Additionally, it must be said that numerous healthcare suppliers are not for empowering breathing in smoke into the lungs in any capacity whatsoever. Tar and other waste products breathed in into the lungs and throat, can aggravate and dry the defensive mucous layers, expanding the danger of disease. Also, the smell of cannabis smoke is observable and thought about hostile to a few.

Disintegrating or "vaping" is a prevalent method for breathing in cannabis (just as tobacco):

This includes preheating a disintegrating gadget to suggested temperature, embeddings a modest quantity of cannabis bloom into the "vape" and afterward breathing in.

Advantages: disintegrating cannabis gives moment alleviation (like smoking), remember the time factor required to warmth up the vaporizer. Vaping doesn't disturb the mucous layers of the throat and lungs as much as smoking.

Disadvantages: Vaping gadgets will in general be expensive; the procedure of vaping for the unpracticed can be testing or cumbersome just as the exceptional impacts for those not certain what's in store. The smell of cannabis smoke is less yet still present.

Edibles: Cannabis is added to common sweet top choices like brownies, treats, confections, dessert, and chewable (like gum). This can be a favored method to ingest for kids and more established grown-ups.

Advantages: edibles are a satisfying method to ingest cannabis, particularly for the individuals who incline toward not to breathe in smoke; no exceptional hardware is required and no smell of smoke is available.

Disadvantages: palatable structures take additional time before the cannabis impact is observable; in this way dosing can be all the more testing. When the impact is felt it very well may be more extreme than foreseen. Like any oral medicine, it ought to be kept far from small kids and pets to avoid unplanned ingestion.

Tinctures: Type of cannabis disintegrated in liquor that can be set on the skin or taken by mouth by putting drops under the tongue or adding to a cup of hot refreshment; once in a while comes in splash structure. Requires progressive dosing to abstain from taking excessively, too early (dependable guideline: start low, go moderate)

Advantages: quicker acting than edibles, yet more slow than breathed in; mellow taste; simple to manage or take.

Disadvantages: less exorbitant when little portions required, all the more expensive with higher dosing necessities.

Oils/Concentrates: concentrates of cannabis infused into cooking oils, like olive oil or coconut oil, which is then cooked into nourishments.

Advantages: Can be effectively be added to most loved dinners and treats; can be used with people, similar to those with Alzheimer, who can't comprehend its use or would oppose taking different types of cannabis or drugs of any sort.

Disadvantages: Like edibles.

Topicals: Salves, creams or fixes applied to the skin; most usually used for agony issue, where the topical can be set over the region of torment, for example, joint inflammation, fibromyalgia (trigger focuses) and musculoskeletal torment.

Advantages: Moisturizers/creams give quick beginning, and fleeting help contrasted with patches that give more slow beginning yet longer alleviation. A few people use a mix of creams/salves and fix application to amplify beginning and length of impact.

Disadvantages: Neighborhood hypersensitive response to fix glue/material or restricting specialist in cream/salve has been accounted for.

Different structures (less regularly used): Suppositories, capsules, squeezing (cannabis infused beverages), eating plant leaves.

Much the same as any help with discomfort choice, cannabis may fill in as a key segment of one individual's torment toolbox and not for another. It is definitely not a one size fits all treatment alternative. This is a choice that ought to be talked about with your healthcare supplier before searching out an authorized marijuana prescriber and gadget. On the off chance that you are as of now taking narcotics for relief from discomfort, see whether you will be required to decrease before cannabis is begun. Before having a talking about with your healthcare supplier, be certain you have gotten your work done.

Check laws and guidelines on medical marijuana in your state and network as they differ. Some different territories to address are:

Will medical marijuana influence your capacity to work and perform anticipated obligations?

Will your activity be secure or is there a danger of employment misfortune if medical marijuana is legitimately recommended?

Is there a danger of losing business related trusted status because of medical marijuana use?

What do you have to know whether you traverse state lines or outside the U.S. while utilizing medical marijuana?

What are the buying rules and confinements in the event that you travel for business or diversion out of state or outside the U.S?

CANNABIS PHENOTYPE AND GENOTYPE

In some cases, you discover a cannabis strain so great, you can't resist the urge to return to the experience each time the open door presents itself. One day you may be amazed to find another cluster of Blue Dream looks in no way like the one you last attempted: what was before a lance formed blossom currently resembles a thick bulb of precious stone trichomes. It's a similar strain, so what's with the fluctuation?

Two things impact the basic development of some random cannabis plant: hereditary qualities and condition.

The plant's hereditary cosmetics, additionally called a genotype, goes about as an outline for development: it permits a range of physical conceivable outcomes, yet it is dependent upon the earth to prompt these attributes. The physical articulation of a genotype is alluded to as a phenotype, which is just characterized as the characteristics that nature hauls out from the plant's hereditary code. Everything from shading, shape, smell, and gum production are influenced by the earth.

This manual for cannabis hereditary qualities will help you through the development of the cannabis plant, from its antique beginnings through the present modern development. Before its finish, you will comprehend that there are in fact characterizing attributes for each strain, yet each plant is as extraordinary as a snowflake as it interestingly communicates qualities as indicated by its nursery condition.

THE EARLIEST CANNABIS SPECIES

Cannabis is an antiquated plant with roots everywhere throughout the world. The soonest species are thought to have developed in the bumpy Hindu Kush area of Pakistan, while others later multiplied in tropical atmospheres. These most punctual assortments, called landrace strains, are viewed as the precious stones of cannabis hereditary qualities. A large number of long stretches of adjustment enabled these strains to express their absolute best qualities for a particular geological area. These territories are what raisers like DJ Short call "sweet spots."

Our short, sap overwhelming indicas populated scopes between 30 to 50 degrees, while the tall, slow-developing sativas normally estate in central areas around 30 degrees scope. These assorted natural surroundings adapted a bright cluster of cannabis assortments, each with its very own long-standing history.

CANNABIS IN THE GREAT INDOORS

Cannabis reproducing took a significant turn starting during the 1970s and 80s when government hostile to cannabis opinions crested, driving development from nature to underground. Indoor gardens, raised by soil, electric lights, and hydroponic frameworks, produce a main part of the cannabis found in the market today. While little uncertainty astonishingly developed strains have been developed inside, specialists will concur that the conventional, unnatural condition can just bring out such a large amount of the plant's potential.

Narrowing decent variety significantly further, producers during this time were fundamentally propelled by THC substance and specifically picked this trademark over other significant concoction constituents like CBD. Disregarding this lost lavishness, we see incredible fluctuation in the plant's phenotypic articulation: supplements, temperature, the sum and point of light, soil type, photoperiod length, time of gather, and the separation between the plant and light source are among the numerous conditions that influence the plant's qualities. Certain conditions may cajole sativa-or indica-like characteristics, so as much as we love arranging strains here at Leafly, we need to recognize that a strain's qualities are not really set in hereditary stone.

THE AGE OF HYBRIDIZATION

Connected at the hip with the indoor develop transformation came hybridized strains, an intermixing of worldwide indigenous assortments. This is the point at which the sativa met the indica, starting a consistently spreading tree of hybrid posterity. Cultivators appreciated indicas for their pitch covered buds and short blooming periods, the two of which are desired characteristics for business production.

In the event that we consider indicas and sativas as falling on furthest edges of the hereditary range, it gets conceivable to envision the extent of phenotypic articulation. Take Blue Dream for instance: a cross between the indica Blueberry and sativa Haze, Blue Dream may think about attributes anyplace the range between its folks, contingent upon how it was raised. This is the reason we may now and then observe an indica-like phenotype of Blue Dream when we expect a sativa. That isn't to say strains are eccentric hereditary special cases; rather, we just shouldn't be astounded when a strain doesn't fit splendidly inside an unmitigated box. Once more, it is conceivable to coax sativa or indica qualities with explicit conditions in a controlled nursery.

Because of hybridization, we have a for all intents and purposes boundless choice of strains to choose from and even energetic strain gatherers will consistently have new hybrids to pursue. Expert focused cultivators may grieve the loss of unique cannabis hereditary qualities; however, many still commit themselves to their restoration. Not exclusively would their recovery make for a more extravagant recreational market, 'antiquated' strains could tremendously affect cannabis as medicine. We trust that as political obstructions fall over like dominoes, the agricultural craft of cannabis development will have the option to sprout all-inclusive by and by.

Really, cannabis rearing is turning out to be more science than workmanship, the impacts of which can be used for everything from torment management to fiber making. Tragically, preclusion has carried with it no shortage of negative symptoms, including an absence of logical examination and distribution about the plant. Simultaneously, the more we find out about cannabis, the more we're starting to understand that things we once thought to be genuine are in reality bogus. A raiser keen on creating a plant with smooth impacts, for instance, may cross two assortments ordinarily alluded to as "indicas," just to locate those two "indicas" contain much more THC than they would have suspected.

Behind these misinterpretations is a basic idea that we've just barely started examining in cannabis: hereditary qualities. In this post, we'll spread some significant ideas and learnings in cannabis hereditary qualities and see how understanding cannabis hereditary qualities can assume a basic job in reproducing that ideal cultivar.

THE BASICS: DEBUNKING THE INDICA VERSUS SATIVA BINARY

The best spot to begin is with the manner in which the vast majority think with regards to arranging cannabis: indica and sativa. Regular terminology places these ordered groupings into a sort of parallel: "sativa" assortments are restricted leafed, tall, lean, and invigorating, while "indica" assortments are expansive leaf, short, ragged and calming.

As we test and find out about these assortments, in any case, we're discovering that the inverse can be valid: tight leaf assortments regularly have calming impacts and wide leaf assortments can be invigorating. So how would you know what an assortment is or what it does? Extremely, the best way to appropriately characterize assortments is to know the chemotype, the cannabinoid and terpene profile, alongside the genotype, it's one of kind hereditary cosmetics.

GENOTYPE VERSUS PHENOTYPES

Genotype depends on the DNA of a living being. Cannabis is diploid, implying that it acquires two duplicates of every quality, one duplicate from each parent. Consequently, the genotype for a quality of intrigue depends on the blend of the two duplicates.

Phenotypes are the noticeable qualities or attributes of a plant that are dictated by genotype and physical condition (counting however not restricted to temperature, moistness, and development rehearses). A few phenotypes — like leaf shape and bloom shading can be seen, though others —, for example, the chemotype of a plant (the concoction phenotype, similar to terpene profile and cannabinoid strength) — must be estimated.

Cannabis hereditary qualities work likewise: one parent plant might be expansive leafed with low degrees of THC, while the other is thin leafed with significant levels of THC. Their youngsters — the seeds — will contain hereditary qualities from the two guardians, and just a portion of those characteristics will communicate when the plant really develops. This is the reason the morphology of the plant, or the manner in which it looks is definitely not an adequate sign of its synthetic substance. Nor, in any case, is a hereditary quality, even clones of precisely the same plant may convey what needs be contrastingly relying upon how they are developed. For instance, a clone raised in an indoor developing office may deliver diverse morphology and chemotype levels than one become outside. Thus, indistinguishable twins may not be superbly indistinguishable: one might be brought into the world with a mole on their cheek, or they may create various physiologies on the off chance that they experience childhood in various situations or have diverse eating and exercise propensities. Along these lines, even precisely the same genotype can deliver various phenotypes.

CHARACTERIZING CANNABIS SATIVA

Understanding that indica and sativa aren't really a paired and that there is, rather, a universe of hereditary assorted variety, prompts a truly significant inquiry: what, at that point, is Cannabis sativa? Are there genuinely different cannabis species?

Here is where hereditary qualities can assist us with finding the appropriate response: through looking at DNA between a large number of tests, we can start to reveal some insight into the connections between various cultivars of cannabis, just as the species limit.

STRAINS OF CANNABIS – INDICA VERSUS SATIVA VERSUS HYBRID

Alright, so now we should discuss these various strains of weed, where they originate from, the distinction between the plants and their development, and what their consequences for the human body are.

SOURCES

The words Indica and Sativa were both acquainted in the eighteenth century with depict the two fundamental kinds of cannabis strains. These are cannabis Indica and cannabis Sativa. The term cannabis Indica was instituted by Jean-Baptiste Lamarck, and this was initially used to portray marijuana for the most part found in India which is high in psychoactive properties, where it was developed and gathered basically for fiber, seeds, and the production of hashish (increasingly here on the distinction among hash and weed). The term cannabis Sativa was authored via Carl Linneaus and was initially used to depict marijuana plants developed in Europe and Western Asia, where it was collected fundamentally for fiber and seeds, yet additionally for its different properties. Since the eighteenth century, there have been numerous newfound and hereditarily adjusted strains of marijuana, with hybrid strains, which are goes among Sativa and Indica, not being made until numerous years after the fact.

Something which is critical to note with regards to the contrasts between Sativa, Indica, and hybrid weed strains is that they easily affect the human body. At the end of the day, these three fundamental sorts of weed impact you in various manners when smoked, disintegrated, or eaten.

Cannabis Indica is for the most part an evening weed and is best smoked or eaten when you have dealt with the entirety of your obligations regarding the day. Indica strains are known for the accompanying impacts on the human body:

- Extraordinary for mental unwinding.

- Assists with muscle unwinding.

- Diminishes sickness.

- Helps increment hunger.

- Helps decline intense and serious agony.

- Expands dopamine — alleviates pressure and discouragement.

- Causes supposed "love seat lock" — best for evening use.

Then again, cannabis Sativa is generally a greater amount of an invigorating kind of marijuana which most would consider best for daytime use. The impacts of cannabis Sativa on the human body incorporate the accompanying:

- Incredible for assuaging uneasiness.

- Useful for calming pressure.

- Helps increment serotonin – controls state of mind.

- Builds innovativeness and center, in a specific way.

- Functions admirably for constant agony.

- Will in general be genuinely invigorating – useful for daytime use.

- Remember that hybrid cannabis strains, due to being a blend of Sativa and Indica strains, can contain a specific level of these properties.

This will rely upon the level of the kinds of weed included when making the Hybrid strains. A few cross breeds can be completely adjusted among Indica and Sativa, some can be Indica prevailing, and some can be Sativa predominant.

PLANT APPEARANCE AND GROWTH

Something different which is important here is that Sativa and Indica strains appear to be unique when they are being developed. At the end of the day, Indica weed plants appear to be unique from Sativa weed plants, and they have somewhat extraordinary development cycle qualities as well. Remember that crossover marijuana strains can extraordinarily vary as far as the plant appearance and development qualities, and it truly depends whether the half breed is a Sativa prevailing, Indica predominant, or a decent strain.

The appearance and development attributes of cannabis Sativa plants incorporate the accompanying:

Cannabis Sativa plants will in general be very tall with genuinely limited leaves. These plants will in general have a genuinely long blossoming cycle, so they take somewhat long to develop and prepare for collect Cannabis Sativa plants are typically most appropriate for development in warm atmospheres which have a long developing season.

The appearance and development qualities of cannabis Indica plants incorporate the accompanying:

Cannabis Indica plants will in general be shorter in stature and bushier than Sativa plants, and have a lot of more extensive leaves. Cannabis Indica plants have a shorter blossoming cycle than Sativa plants, by as much as 2 or 3 weeks, and in this manner are snappier to develop and get the chance to reap. Cannabis Indica plants are most appropriate for marginally cooler atmospheres with to some degree shorter developing seasons.

DIFFERENCE BETWEEN THC AND CBD STRAINS

Something that is likewise imperative to note here is the contrast among CBD and THC. What you cannot deny is that marijuana contains something known as cannabinoids. The weed plant has many synthetic substances in it. The primary segments which cause the real and mental impacts are terpenes and cannabinoids. The two principle and most basic cannabinoids are THC and CBD, and they can have altogether different consequences for the body and psyche.

THC DOMINANT MARIJUANA STRAINS

THC represents Tetrahydrocannabinol. These are the strains which are typically picked by individuals who need an unwinding and calming strain for evening use. They are extraordinary for treating extreme agony, an absence of hunger, sickness, tension, gloom, and that's only the tip of the iceberg. This is the sort of weed that gives you a solid and euphoric head high, will in general make you genuinely drained, and it causes hunger too. This is the sort of weed that gives you the munchies.

CBD DOMINANT MARIJUANA STRAINS

CBD represents cannabidiol. This is really a non-inebriating compound. As such, it doesn't create a euphoric head high. It as a rule doesn't cause tiredness or yearning, in any event on the off chance that you just smoke a touch of it. This is a decent strain to go with to ease ceaseless torment, to move innovativeness, to diminish aggravation, and that's only the tip of the iceberg. It's a decent decision to go with in the event that you need help from different side effects, however don't need that yearning actuating, love seat locking head high. Something significant here is that there is a misguided judgment that CBD overwhelming strains are really invigorating. People, Sativa isn't a similar thing as a Red Bull or some espresso. It simply doesn't work that way. While CBD overwhelming strains won't make you as worn out, or cause you to wear out as awful as Indica substantial strains, they will inevitably still make you somewhat drained, simply less so than Indica.

ADJUSTED CBD AND THC MARIJUANA STRAINS

Marijuana strains which contain a parity of THC and CBD is a decision which numerous individuals will in general go with. These strains will in general produce a mellow to respectably euphoric head high, a touch of appetite, and are really useful for sleep deprivation, while they additionally contain a specific measure of manifestation help. This truly relies upon the harmony among THC and CBD, and can change incredibly starting with one strain then onto the next.

Sativa Versus Indica And CBD Versus THC – A Common Misconception Cannabis Plant Appearance

What is entrancing to note is that for a long time, it was acknowledged that most Indica strains contain more CBD than THC, and that Sativa strains contained more THC than CBD. Regardless, this isn't commonly the circumstance in any way shape or form. As a rule, if you somehow happened to inspect 100 marijuana strains, the outcome ought to be that Indica strains by and large contain all the more calming THC, while most Sativa strains contain more CBD. This is significant on the grounds that this has been an extremely huge misguided judgment for quite a while. Despite that fact, what you likewise need to know is that the profiles of Indica, Sativa, and hybrid strains have changed and broadened after some time.

Presently, it is never again exact to state one way or the other. Some Indica strains may be truly elevated in CBD or THC, however not the other, or both, and this goes for Sativa and hybrid strains as well. In spite of the fact that the Indica, Sativa, and hybrid characterizations still stay famous and broadly utilized today, they are not constantly exact regarding educating the shopper regarding the genuine THC and CBD includes in them. This is the reason you have to investigate every individual strain before settling on an acquiring choice.

A NOTE ON TERPENES

As we referenced over, another of the fundamental mixes found in all marijuana strains are terpenes. In the event that you didn't have the foggiest idea, terpenes are a kind of sweet-smelling compound created by most leafy foods, and indeed, marijuana is a blooming plant. You will discover terpenes contained in numerous sweet-smelling blossoms, lavender, citrus organic products, peppers, and indeed, cannabis as well. Terpenes are the principle contributing element to that fruity, fancy, citrusy, berry-like, and numerous different aromas and tastes which your strain of marijuana may highlight. Various strains of weed contain various terpenes, and there are a wide range of sorts of terpenes to go around.

There are a couple of extremely regular terpenes found in marijuana. One of these is linalool, which is known to be unwinding. Another regular terpene found in cannabis is pinene, which highlights a greater amount of a cautioning property. Be that as it may, the truth is that making sense of which terpenes because which impacts is truly difficult to measure. None the less, it merits inspecting the most well-known terpenes found in marijuana;

- **Alpha Pinene** – This terpene scents like pine or pine needles, it will in general increment sharpness and memory maintenance, and can be utilized for treating asthma, agony, irritation, and nervousness.

- **Myrcene** – This terpene has a musky, natural, and home grown like smell, and regularly scents like cloves or cardamom. Myrcene will in general have an unwinding, quieting, and lounge chair locking impact. It is a decent enemy of oxidant, it assists with a sleeping disorder, agony, and irritation.

- **Limonene** – This terpene has a very citrusy smell and flavor, and it hoists your state of mind and helps with pressure alleviation. It tends to be utilized to treat uneasiness, stress, gloom, irritation, and agony.

- **Caryophyllene** – This terpene has a zesty and peppery smell and taste, regularly woody too. This is an extraordinary terpene for stress alleviation and is regularly known to help with agony, tension, and gloom.

- **Linalool** – This terpene has an extremely extravagant smell and taste. It has the impacts of sedation and mind-set improvement. It very well may be utilized to help treat sleep deprivation, torment, melancholy, tension, stress, and irritation.

- **Humulene** – This terpene has a hoppy, natural, and woody flavor. It's best known for having calming properties.

- **Ocimene** – Ocimene is a terpene which has a sweet, woody, and natural like smell and flavor. It is outstanding for having hostile to septic, against contagious, and against viral properties, and it is referred to as a decongestant too.

- **Terpinolene** – This terpene has a flower, piney, and home-grown aroma and flavor. It is unwinding, it fills in as an enemy of oxidant, and is soothing in nature.

MOST POPULAR STRAINS OF CANNABIS

Here, we just want to list some of the most popular and widely purchased strains of Cannabis in all 3 categories, Sativa, Indica, and hybrid. These strains are definitely worth trying out.

SATIVA:

- Acapulco Gold

- Allen Wrench

- Amnesia

- Chocolope

- Cinex

- Dirty Girl

- Durban Poison

- Ghost Train Haze

- Grapefruit

- Green Crack

- Harlequin

- Sweet Skunk

- Jack Herer

- Kali Mist

- Maui Wowie

- Purple Haze

- Sour Diesel

- Lemon Haze

- Silver Haze

Indica:

- Afghani

- Blueberry

- Bubba Kush

- G13

- Granddaddy Purple

- Green Ape

- Hindu Kush

- Lavender

- Master Kush

- Northern Lights

- Presidential OG

- Purple Urkle

HYBRID:

- ACDC

- Ak-47

- Banana OG

- Blue Dream

- Catatonic

- Chernobyl

- Cherry Pie

- Cinderella 99

- Double Dream

- Dutch Treat

- Fruity Pebbles

- Gelato

- Jillybean

- Juicy Fruit

- Larry OG

- Lodi Dodi

- Mango Kush

- OG Kush

- Permafrost

- Pineapple Express

- Pink Kush

- Snoop's Dream

- Sour Tsunami

- Space Queen

- Tahoe OG

- Trainwreck

- UK Cheese

- White Fire OG

- White Widow

PICKING THE RIGHT CANNABIS STRAIN FOR YOU

Presently you know pretty much everything there is to think about the different strains and sorts of weed. Allows simply emphasize some central matters of center with regards to picking the correct sort of marijuana for you. What would you like to escape your smoking, disintegrating, or edibles experience? Do you need help with discomfort, tension and sorrow management, do you need something to make you hungry, do you experience the ill effects of sleep deprivation? On the off chance that you are utilizing marijuana for medical conditions, you have to pick the correct strain, with the best possible CBD and THC content for the activity.

What scents and smells to you like? Indeed, this is alluding to the terpenes. You may like weed that is greater fruity, woody, nutty, natural, citrusy, or whatever else. Consider the terpene and flavor profile of the marijuana strain being referred to before settling on a decision. It is safe to say that you are smoking, vaping, or eating edibles during the day or around evening time? As a rule, Sativa won't make you as worn out or ravenous as Indica strains as well, something essential to remember whether you plan on being dynamic during the day or need a decent night's rest. Keep in mind that THC is the thing that creates a euphoric head high, while CBD generally doesn't deliver a lot of a high by any means. CBD is best for side effect help, while THC is incredible for making you feel high.

CONCEIVABLE SIDE EFFECTS OF THC MARIJUANA DOMINANT STRAINS

Before we wrap up for the afternoon, something you should know is that for certain individuals, strains which are exceptionally overwhelming in THC can cause some symptoms. Presently, this is definitely not a slam dunk, as everyone responds in an unexpected way. Sadly, this is a preliminary by blunder sort of thing, and you won't ever truly know how you will respond to THC substantial weed until you attempt it for yourself. Notwithstanding, basically a mess of THC can possibly create some entirely serious reactions in individuals, and truly, there are individuals who are adversely affected by it. On the off chance that you need tension and help with discomfort, however can't deal with a great deal of THC, you should go with a CBD overwhelming strain, or possibly one that is well-adjusted between the two.

A portion of the conceivable reactions of THC substantial marijuana strains incorporate the accompanying:

- Tension

- Melancholy

- Suspicion (One of the most widely recognized reactions in numerous individuals)

- Outrageous laziness – love seat lock

- Cerebral pains

- Tipsiness

- Wooziness

- Dry and irritated eyes

Presently you should know essentially everything about the contrasts between Indica, Sativa, and hybrid marijuana strains. To individuals who are not customary cannabis clients, this may sound somewhat trifling. Be that as it may, regardless of anything else, there are some huge contrasts between the principle strains and sorts of weed. Realizing the distinctions will assist you with picking the correct one dependent on what sort of impacts and results you are hoping to accomplish.

GREENHOUSE CULTIVATION OF CANNABIS FOR SEEDS USED IN PRODUCTION OF CANNABIS PHARMACY OIL

With any greenhouse structure, it is imperative to remember the end reason directly from the beginning. Greenhouses are worked to give your yield, whatever it is, with the perfect developing condition. On the off chance that you are developing annuals or perennials you may need to assemble some adaptability in your greenhouse structure to oblige various plants with various climatic needs. On the off chance that you are just developing tomatoes, your greenhouse can be structured worked to concentrate altogether on boosting production efficiencies and yield of that plant.

Marijuana is a controlled substance, so expecting you have paid some dues to be granted one of the pined for cultivation licenses, it is far-fetched that your marijuana greenhouse will develop any plants outside the cannabis family. So, for developing marijuana plants, you need to concentrate on the perfect condition for cannabis.

The 4 Stages of Growth for Cannabis Production Affect How You Zone Your Greenhouse

- Zone 1: Marijuana mother plants

- Zone 2: Marijuana clones (cuttings)

- Zone 3: Marijuana in the vegetative stage

- Zone 4: Marijuana in the bloom stage

PLAN FOR EXPANSION FROM THE START

On the off chance that you are as of now developing harvests effectively in a greenhouse, it is anything but difficult to concentrate your cannabis business energies on the yield developing side. Be that as it may, dismissing this all in all new business with various clients and distinctive circulation directs will get you in a tough situation. Start your cannabis greenhouse measured for your not so distant future client requests yet in view of adaptability to suit your more drawn out term business objectives. We work with cultivators everywhere throughout the world structuring greenhouses for different stage extension plans. Some additional time toward the start can spare you long stretches of migraines and extra expenses not far off.

PARITY PRODUCTION EFFICIENCIES

Marijuana producers are accustomed to developing in littler spaces than most business cultivators. Greenhouse structures and modern plant developing innovation offer huge production advantages contrasted with run of the mill indoor developing. Be that as it may, where huge zones increment production productivity, they additionally increment harvest chance from ailment or pervasion spreading. At the point when you consider the financial estimation of your marijuana crop, and perhaps the medical basic of giving reliable medicine to your patients, there is a sensible tradeoff between production scale zones and detachment portioning.

Zone division can without much of a stretch be accomplished with inside peak dividers and sidewalls, an appropriately structured greenhouse warming and cooling framework and great natural controls. Power outage blinds (otherwise called light hardship screens), water system, and fertigation frameworks are altogether

66

structured by greenhouse industry specialists to be midway controlled for numerous zones.

BUILDING THE IDEAL ENVIRONMENT

- **Geographic area:** I can't overemphasize the significance of this point. Not every greenhouse maker or cannabis developing specialists have involvement with various land areas. Numerous individuals will attempt to sell you the greenhouse that has been effective in Colorado, however in the event that you are in Southern California, Puerto Rico, or Alaska, the greenhouse you need will be altogether different. Your outside temperature vacillations, wind speeds, stickiness levels, snow loads, and light levels all factor into what gear and the style of structure that is best for you and your yield.

- **Inside greenhouse temperature:** Cannabis like numerous harvests likes various temperatures at various stages of development. As a speculation you need your greenhouse temperatures between 65 to 85° F. Your greenhouse warming and cooling frameworks need to consider the temperature needs and controls for each zone. Unpracticed experts may disclose to you that you don't require as a lot of warming on the grounds that the lights produce a great deal of warmth, yet as you will find in the segments underneath, cannabis ordinarily needs just 18 or 12 hours of light, so your coldest evening time temperatures will in any case commonly have no lights on by any stretch of the imagination.

- **Overseeing stickiness inside a cannabis greenhouse:** We as a whole know the impacts stickiness has on plants. To an extreme, and your welcome illness, excessively little and you dry out the plant and prevent development. Similarly, as with any harvest, knowing the dampness that the plant flourishes in is significant when planning a greenhouse. While cannabis in the vegetative stage really loves a higher moistness level, it leans towards lower stickiness when in blossom. Greenhouse producers who comprehend this can assist you with building adaptability into your greenhouse structures. There are a few dehumidification units available, and for zones requiring the capacity to include dampness moistening frameworks can be included into the greenhouse structure.

- **Ventilation proposals for greenhouses tie into temperature and moistness needs:** Greenhouse ventilation separates into two fundamental classifications: 1) common ventilation spreads rooftop vents, sidewall vents and rollup sides, and 2) constrained air ventilation requires mechanical frameworks like fumes fans, and in some cases cooling cushions. Kindly note that cooling cushions are not a decent choice for high dampness districts. Notwithstanding ventilation to expel tourist from inside the greenhouse, most greenhouse cultivators put wind stream fans inside the greenhouse to flow air development which is useful for keeping healthy plants. Greenhouse makers can furnish you with a greenhouse plan design demonstrating fan areas that streamline wind stream coverage.

- **Altering lighting levels will build yields in a cannabis greenhouse**: Perhaps the greatest advantage that greenhouse developing ideas over indoor developing is that greenhouse plants profit by common daylight. Not exclusively does daylight normally give the plants what they have to develop, it doesn't cost the cultivator any cash to control. Having said that, when cannabis is in the vegetative state it performs best with around 18 hours of light. Therefore, we prescribe greenhouse cultivators incorporate supplemental lighting in their cannabis greenhouse arrangement. Ensure your greenhouse lighting plans fulfill all year production on the off chance that you need to upgrade yields.

- **Blossoming cannabis needs power outage.** While the vegetative stage appreciates more prominent light levels, for blooming longer times of murkiness are wanted. Guaranteeing 12 hours of continuous murkiness inside your greenhouse will constrain the marijuana plants to bloom as per your production plan. This is best accomplished by using power outage window ornament innovation, otherwise called light hardship in the marijuana business. Power outage has been ordinarily utilized in production greenhouses for quite a long time for poinsettias, kalanchoes, mums and other crops that profit by photoperiod changes. Power outage blinds can cover level rooftop zones running bracket to support on canal associated greenhouses, or they can be slanted to pursue the rooftop line of detached greenhouses. Make sure to cover sidewalls and entryway openings, and at GGS we give light traps to debilitate fans too.

- **Cannabis plants flourish with CO_2 advancement:** On the off chance that you are utilizing a high temp water warming framework CO_2 can be pulled off the boiler. In different cases you may wish to utilize fluid CO_2 to portion your cannabis crop. This is a zone best examined with greenhouse warming specialists like our sister organization Niagrow Systems. Extra contemplations incorporate associating your greenhouse to distribution center and office offices for bundling, delivery, and other bolster capacities. There are other exceptional necessities for cannabis that you won't have experienced with run of the mill plant crops, for example, drying rooms and vaults. Work with an organization that has the mastery to support you.

- **Supplement:** Supplements are taken up from the soil by roots. Supplement soil corrections (composts) are included when the soil supplements are drained. Manures can be compound or natural, fluid or powder, and as a rule contain a blend of fixings. Business composts indicate the degrees of NPK (nitrogen, phosphorus, and potassium). When all is said in done, cannabis needs more N than P and K during all life stages. The nearness of auxiliary supplements (calcium, magnesium, sulfur) is suggested. Micronutrients (for example iron, boron, chlorine, manganese, copper, zinc, molybdenum) infrequently show as insufficiencies. Since cannabis' supplement needs differ generally relying upon the assortment, they are typically dictated by experimentation and manures are applied sparingly to abstain from consuming the plant.

Concerning gathering, one of the most empowering things you can choose to accumulate are cannabis seeds. These questionable little beans are one of the most genetically planned normal products available, likely only to some degree behind roses. The astonishing qualities alongside the sheer number of various strains of seed accessible make them one of the most fascinating and most overwhelming accumulations to begin. One of the missions a few gatherers embrace is to attempt to locate their ideal cannabis seed. Each unique strain holds an alternate arrangement of ascribes which will join to give you the ideal seed that matches your taste.

THC: THC means 'Tetrahydrocannabinol'. This is the principle psychoactive part found in a completely developed cannabis plant and when you search for seeds you will see the THC rate recorded. While your seeds won't contain any genuine THC, each strain has been intended to dependably deliver a plant that will have this degree of THC. In the event that you are fortunate enough to live in a nation where developing cannabis is legitimate you will have the option to test it out. On the off chance that you are not, you should manage with your ideal seed having the capacity to deliver certain degrees of THC.

Yield: Another thing you may get a kick out of the chance to think about your cannabis seed is how a lot of cannabis it could make on the off chance that it was lawful to develop it. Yield is typically estimated in grams and is worked out by the normal yield found by the reproducer. In the event that you like to realize your seed could deliver a high return this is a credit you may get a kick out of the chance to take a gander at.

Strain: Choosing a strain isn't just about the imperative measurements however. You find genuinely comparative THC and yield levels on various cannabis seeds so you have to pick a strain you like. A respectable technique to do this is to look at ones that have won bona fide distinctions for quality. The most regarded of which is certainly the High Times Cannabis Cup. Consistently they judge what seed bank and what individual cannabis seed is the best of the year. Feminized seeds are apparently the most de rigueur at the present time.

PRODUCTION OF CANNABIS

PHARMACY OIL

Nowadays, CBD oil business is on the ascent. Actually, the market will appreciate fast development as there is a great deal of interest for the product. A couple of individuals don't have the foggiest thought regarding the wellspring of the oil. Everything considered, CBD is short for Cannabidiol. Essentially, the oil is removed from a plant and is helpful for individuals with stress, joint pain and numerous different conditions. On the off chance that you need a couple of strong systems to assist you with beginning and develop your business by selling this oil, you might need to peruse this guide.

- **Register your Business:** First, you have to get a license. As it were, you have to get your business enlisted. This applies regardless of whether you need to open an on the web or physical store. Individuals want to purchase from an enlisted merchant so as to dodge con artists. Purchasing unique products is everybody's worry.

- **Dispatch a Website:** Once you have your business enrolled, your best course of action is to make a site to advertise your products. Ensure your site is average enough. For this, you have to decide on a dependable web designer.

- **Pick a Merchant Processor:** You have to search for a dependable shipper processor. This is significant in the event that you need to get installment for your product deals. While it's legitimate to keep up a CBD oil business, various merchant processors think this kind of business incorporates a huge amount of danger.

- Keep the Law: Once you have picked a trader, your best course of action is to adhere to the government laws. As it were, you should keep the laws identified with the clearance of medical and recreational cannabis products. Thinking about all, you would incline toward not to violate any laws while your business is creating.

- **Run Marketing Campaigns**: Irrespective of the sort of business you run, ensure you find a way to advertise your products. In actuality, marketing is the foundation of any business. With the correct marketing techniques, you can communicate as the need should arise to a great deal of potential clients. The perfect method for marketing your business is by means of Google promotions, blog entries, and different kinds of advertisements. Beside this, you can utilize the intensity of online networking to arrive at much more clients. In any case, to make your web-based life marketing effective, you have to make posts that are locks in. With the help of SEO, you can without quite a bit of a stretch position your site. To answer the request of your customers, you must have a solid customer care organization on your site. Open your Online Store: A straightforward technique for extending your arrangements is to dispatch an online store. You may need to offer a colossal grouping of products through your store. It will be more straightforward for you to build up your customers if you offer a combination of products. All things considered, not all clients like to purchase a similar product. CBD oil is utilized diversely dependent on the kind of condition a patient has.

PRODUCTION AND EXTRACTION OF CBD OIL

Cannabidiol (CBD) is one of numerous normally happening cannabinoid found in the cannabis plant. Both hemp and marijuana can contain CBD, however today CBD products are fundamentally made from hemp. Dissimilar to marijuana which contains a lot of THC, the high prompting compound in cannabis, hemp contains all things considered follow sums.

While there is a developing business sector for smoked hemp blossom, the most well-known approach to devour the gainful phytocompounds is by means of tinctures or containers. So as to be devoured as such, the normally happening mixes in the plant must be separated into oil structure. This oil is then utilized as the essential fixing in these and a lot progressively consumable and topical product.

The technique for extraction and handling of a hemp concentrate can bigly affect the substance, quality, and immaculateness of a given product. In this book, we spread the different techniques for extraction used to make CBD oil from hemp. Continue perusing to find what goes into the making of a CBD product and what sorts of extraction and handling are liked. Hemp has at last been given a definition separate from marijuana. This definition lifts hemp out of the controlled substances act, making the plant and its concentrates lawful. The meaning of hemp is cannabis containing 0.3% or less THC by dry weight. This lawful status and the high-CBD substance of numerous strains has prompted hemp being the essential wellspring of CBD oil extraction for products offered to people in general.

It is conceivable to discover high-CBD products removed from marijuana, yet they are additionally regularly high in THC and in this manner today should be sold as a marijuana product through fitting channels. These products are outside the extent of this book, and any CBD product you find uninhibitedly accessible available to be purchased on the web and in retail locations will be hemp-inferred. This is phenomenal news as it implies there are numerous viable, clean products accessible. This legitimate endorsement has brought forth an undeniably huge number of cultivators and extractors who look to create the most excellent hemp conceivable. Today you'll discover an abundance of products sourced from naturally developed, non-GMO, local hemp plants.

COMPARING CBD OIL EXTRACTION METHODS

As we talked about in the introduction, the hemp plant first needs to experience an extraction procedure all together for the plant mixes to be changed into one of the numerous products accessible available today. The general thought of hemp extraction is that a dissolvable is gone through plant material so as to separate out the dynamic mixes in the mass plant materials. The subsequent cannabinoids, terpenes, and other plant mixes like chlorophyll are then gathered as oil and further prepared before advancing into a final result.

The accompanying techniques are for the most part normally used to make the different ranges of CBD oil concentrates found available today. Every strategy conveys impediments and advantages which we spread underneath:

Supercritical CO2 Extraction-CO2 extraction is broadly viewed as an incredible technique used to make CBD-rich removes. This extraction technique puts carbon dioxide under high weight while keeping up a low temperature. The gas is changed into a fluid because of the weight and afterward went through the plant material with up to a 90% extraction proficiency. The subsequent concentrates an exceptionally focused, absolutely unadulterated oil separate. This procedure requires costly hardware and experienced administrators. Along these lines, the subsequent oil is regularly more extravagant for the end buyer however empowers the most excellent products to be delivered.

- **Ethanol Extraction**: When contrasted with CO2 extraction, ethanol extraction is a lower-cost technique, yet utilized by numerous organizations available today. Notwithstanding the lower cost, this extraction strategy can at present be utilized to make top notch removes however it might require more mastery and post-extraction handling. This extraction strategy uses a liquor dissolvable - most generally ethanol. Ethanol is 'By and large Regarded as Safe (GRAS)' by the FDA. It is normally utilized as a nourishment additive and added substance found in numerous products at the market. Ethanol is a polar dissolvable which means it will blend in with water and break down water-solvent particles notwithstanding the ideal cannabis mixes. Chlorophyll is one of the intensifies that ethanol will co-remove alongside the cannabinoid filled oil. The outcome is a dim hued oil with a severe and lush flavor.

The chlorophyll can be expelled from the oil utilizing post-extraction sifting techniques, however the procedure can likewise evacuate a portion of the cannabinoids bringing about a lower quality CBD oil product. Some ethanol extractors refer to that the water-solvent part extraction can be alleviated by utilizing cold extraction temperatures. Accepting an accomplished administrator, the aftereffect of this extraction strategy can be truly great, even tantamount to CO2 extraction in quality. That being stated, with a less experienced extractor, there is more space for blunder and probability for dissolvable tainting or lower quality finished result.

- **Hydrocarbon Extraction**: This early extraction technique was made utilizing a light hydrocarbon dissolvable like to separate cannabis oil. Usually butane, pentane, propane, hexane, isopropyl liquor or CH3)2CO are utilized as solvents. These hydrocarbons have a low boiling point and can be effectively used to extricate CBD oil. This modest and simple technique for extraction accompanies an assortment of issues that make it non-perfect. The subsequent oil generally contains a lower convergence of terpenes and cannabinoids like CBD and a higher centralization of THC. There is likewise risky buildup that can remain that may meddle with safe capacity. This extraction technique demonstrated to be both hazardous a wasteful and is along these lines once in a while utilized by business CBD organizations today.

- **Lipid Extraction**: One of the lesser-utilized extraction techniques is called lipid extraction. This strategy utilizes the fats, or "lipids", to assimilate and embody the hemp-delivered mixes. Frequently natural coconut oil is utilized in this extraction procedure. Lipid extraction doesn't require the utilization of any brutal solvents or

CO2. It's anything but a well-known strategy for extraction, however you may discover some boutique organizations utilizing it.

After a CBD concentrate is made, there are some extra, discretionary steps that are performed to prepare the product for utilization. Actuating by means of Decarboxylation. The normally happening cannabinoids found in the cannabis plant arrive in a corrosive structure including:

- CBDA (Cannabidiolic corrosive)

- THCA (Tetrahydrocannabinolic corrosive)

- CBGA (Cannabigerolic corrosive)

These 'crude' cannabinoids must be enacted so as to create the ideal particles. For instance, CBDA must be enacted to deliver CBD. At the point when a low-temperature technique like supercritical CO2 extraction is utilized, the first corrosive types of the cannabinoids might be created. So as to initiate these cannabinoids and evacuated the corrosive atom, the CBD concentrate experiences a procedure called decarboxylation. Despite the fact that it sounds extravagant, decarboxylation is basically the warming of a concentrate. Through this warming procedure, the corrosive particle is evacuated and the dynamic compound is delivered. Regardless of being less prevalent, the 'crude' particles are demonstrating guarantee as they interface with the body uniquely in contrast to the 'actuated' or non-corrosive types of these equivalent substances. For instance, THCA is non-psychoactive, while THC is psychoactive. Restricted research and episodic client encounters point to these crude cannabinoid structures giving some interesting helpful benefits. This is driving a few organizations to incorporate the corrosive types of these cannabinoids notwithstanding the enacted non-corrosive structures. All things considered, except if explicitly laid out as a 'crude' product, all CBD products available have been decarboxylated to actuate the mixes.

CLEANSING BY MEANS OF WINTERIZATION

At the point when the oil concentrate was made utilizing high weight or high temperatures, the extraction procedure pulls a wide scope of unsaturated fats, plant materials, chlorophyll, cannabinoids, and terpenoids from the plant material. For concentrates of this sort, there is a discretionary procedure called winterization which attempts to further filter the concentrate and expel the undesirable parts. The way toward winterizing comprises of totally blending the CBD separate in 200 proof liquor and solidifying it medium-term. In the first part of the day the shady blend is prepared for filtration. This procedure is finished by running it through a paper channel into an extraction container. The liquor is expelled from the separated final result through warming until it vanishes. This is made conceivable in light of the fact that the liquor has a lower boiling point than the oil.

HOW CBD ISOLATE IS MADE?

Since you comprehend CBD extraction, it is opportunity to make things a stride further. Today you'll generally discover single-atom CBD confines. In their most perfect structure, these disengages are a crystalline white powder included 99%+ cannabidiol. All different cannabinoids, terpenes, plant materials, oil, and chlorophyll are evacuated in the production of this powder. All that is left is normally sourced CBD precious stones that convey no smell or flavor. This seclude is made by first extricating oil utilizing one of the techniques we talked about above and afterward winterizing. Next, scientists can utilize short way refining or chromatography disengage the individual mixes in the material - for this situation, cannabidiol. For short way refining, this works similarly as winterization as each compound can be disconnected through their extraordinary boiling points.

Consumers regularly discover CBD seclude alluring on the grounds that it is without THC. You ought to get that while seclude is adaptable, products dependent on this sort of concentrate are not as compelling as an oil containing a full or wide range cannabinoid profile. The single-cannabinoid profile is less successful because of the absence of cannabinoid and terpene cooperative energies known as the escort effect. Here at Big Sky Botanicals, we produce a wide range product line that contains a full-range profile of cannabinoids and terpenes with just the THC expelled. Since you see how CBD oil is made, make certain to look at how our products are made which layouts the extraction and preparing strategies we use to make our product line.

CANNABIS PHARMACY OILS AND ITS USAGE

CBD speaks to cannabidiol oil. It is used to treat different appearances notwithstanding the way that its usage is genuinely sketchy. There is moreover some disorder as for how absolutely the oil impacts our bodies. The oil may have medical advantages and such products that have the compound are genuine in various spots today.

GETTING THC AND CBD

CBD is a cannabinoid, a compound found in cannabis plant. The oil contains CBD centers and the usages change fundamentally. In cannabis, the exacerbate that is remarkable is delta 9 tetrahydrocannabinol or THC. It is a working fixing found in marijuana. Marijuana has CBD and THC and both have different effects.

THC alters the mind when one is smoking or cooking with it. This is in light of the fact that it is isolated by heat. As opposed to THC, CBD isn't psychoactive. This infers your point of view doesn't change with use. In any case, critical changes can be noted inside the human body suggesting medical advantages.

SOURCE

Hemp is a bit of the cannabis plant and all around, it isn't dealt with. This is the spot a lot of the CBD is evacuated. Marijuana and hemp start from cannabis sativa, anyway are remarkable. Today, marijuana ranchers are copying plants with the target that they can have high THC levels. Hemp farmers don't need to alter plants and are used to make the CBD oil.

Cannabinoids impact the body by interfacing themselves to different receptors. Some cannabinoids are conveyed by the body and there are the CB1 and CB2 receptors. CB1 receptors are discovered all through the body with a dumbfounding number of them being in the cerebrum. The receptors are liable for attitude, emotions, torment, improvement, coordination, memories, craving, thinking, and various limits. THC impacts these receptors.

Concerning the CB2 receptors, they are transcendently in one's protected structure and impact desolation and disturbance. Regardless of the way that CBD doesn't annex direct here, it manages the body to use cannabinoids more.

THE ADVANTAGES

CBD is productive to human wellbeing in different ways. It is a trademark distress reliever and has quieting properties. Over the counter medications are used for help with distress and by far most lean toward a dynamically regular other choice and this is the spot CBD oil comes in. Research has shown that CBD gives a predominant treatment, especially for people with relentless torment. There is similarly verification that recommend that the use of CBD can be amazingly helpful for any person who is endeavoring to quit smoking and overseeing drug withdrawals. In an appraisal, it was seen that smokers who had inhalers that had CBD would when all is said in done smoke not as much as what was commonplace for them and with no further needing for cigarettes. CBD could be an unfathomable treatment for people with oppression issue particularly to sedatives.

There are various other medical conditions that are bolstered by CBD and they fuse epilepsy, LGA, Dravet issue, seizures, and so on. More research is being coordinated on the effects of CBD in the human body and the results are empowering. The likelihood of doing combating dangerous development and differing pressure issue is moreover being looked. For all of you who are still on the "Basically Say No" brief prevailing fashion, you may acknowledge that hemp seed oil, which is gotten from the seeds of the cannabis plant, is essentially one more course for those darn radicals to get high. In any case, while the blooms this questionable plant are fit for accomplishing delicate mental outings and making everything on FOX News seem, by all accounts, to be entertaining, the seeds and the accommodating oily oils that they contain, will achieve no such thing. In all honesty, hemp seed oil is accepted to be one of the most productive upgrades an individual can take in order to keep up a working and solid lifestyle.

Some time back before administrators and business interests got included, hemp was a noteworthy yield with any advanced and helpful occupations. On the wellbeing front, the seeds of the hemp plant were viewed as a for all intents and purposes immaculate sustenance source, containing 80% of the fundamental unsaturated fats that our bodies need correspondingly as globule destines which is an unprecedented protein that takes after globulin. Hemp oil is viably consumable and contains for all intents and purposes the aggregate of the central unsaturated fats that the body needs in order to stay working fittingly. Present day Research studies have found that taking hemp oil constantly can help fix a hurt insusceptible structure and even switch wasting making it a critical ordinary upgrade for both sickness patients and people with AIDS.

TAKING INTERNALLY CANNABIS OIL CAN:

- Increment essentialness

- Help with engine abilities

- Straightforwardness Arthritis Pain

- Fortify the Immune System

- Treat Tuberculosis

- Reduction Sun Related Damage to the skin

Individuals with conditions brought about by inadequacy in LA (Omega 6) and LNA (Omega 3) can be treated by taking hemp oil since it has those fundamental unsaturated fats (EFA) in adjusted, perfect extents. Hemp seed oil has a low level of Stearic destructive (18:0) which is beneficial for wellbeing since noteworthy degrees of Stearic destructive structure stream blocking clusters in veins and kill the retouching attributes of the EFA's.

THE AMOUNT TO TAKE:

On the consistent schedule you can take 2-4 pastry spoons (up to 50 ml) every day. On account of treatment you can expand the portion up to 150 ml for every day for around 7 days, at that point come back to the ordinary day by day sum. Hemp Seed Oil has a nutty flavor that the vast majority find lovely. It is a perfect added substance to plate of mixed greens dressings, plunges, or cold pasta. It isn't appropriate for singing, since overabundance warmth will extraordinarily decrease a large number of its nurturing benefits. It can in like manner be used remotely to treat skin conditions, for instance, dermatitis. You can think that its numerous health nourishment stores.

There is a colossal issue that exists today with the tremendous number of individuals experiencing joint inflammation in its numerous structures. It is said that well over a large portion of the number of inhabitants in this nation who are more than 60 experience the ill effects of either osteo or rheumatoid joint pain. What the two types of the illness really are I won't go into here, as it is a long and complex subject. Yet, joint pain is a type of irritation which standard medicine seems incapable to address.

Both are brought about by what I call "bone and ligament rock", the bits of bone and ligament which are left in the joints after the body has begun to decline, focusing on the joints each time it moves. This "rock" rubs on the nerve closes, causing torment, while simultaneously making more harm as the "rock" keeps on scouring endlessly a greater amount of the bone and ligament. As such, an endless loop that modern medicine can't resolve. Be that as it may, there are routes in the elective cure field that may, and I am aware of numerous cases that have, had the option to break this circle.

I suggest that an everyday Hemp Oil Capsule, or the fluid slick, which is very delectable, and can be removed a spoon, ought to be viewed as long haul. Hemp Oil originates from hemp seed:

The Most Nutritionally Complete Food Source in The World.

The Essential Fatty Acids in hemp are renowned for their ability to improve cell advancement and organ limit, Hemp Oil is sensible for Vegetarians and Vegans.

There has been a passionate climb in news respect for restorative cannabis in 2013, with gives insights about CNN, ABC, CBS, and neighborhood conveyances about high-cannabidiol cannabis oil effectively controlling the indications of unprecedented epileptic conditions like Dravet issue, Doose issue, immature fits, cortical dysplasia, and that is just a hint of something larger. These diseases can make hundreds countless seizures seven days, while moreover blocking headway in different various ways. For families with adolescents encountering such conditions, the troubles are overwhelming. Due to the very astounding nature of Dravet and related issue, standard pharmaceuticals are unable and as often as possible bother the issues. With no other desire, families have gone to high-CBD cannabis oil, which is showing to work with wonderful suitability.

To clarify, high-CBD cannabis oil is non-psychoactive and clearly extensively more critical than high-THC cannabis oil. Cannabidiol is another cannabinoid in the cannabis plant, like the all the all the more striking psychoactive cannabinoid THC, with essential research prescribing neuroprotectant, anticancer, antidiabetic, threatening to ischemic, antispasmodic, antipsychotic, and antibacterial properties, among others. Additionally, cannabis oil is a sort of concentrate from cannabis. Such oil contains a great deal of concentrated cannabinoids that can be orally ingested rather than smoked, securing the therapeutic blends and empowering them to be passed on through stomach related structure, instead of the respiratory system.

The examination prescribes that CBD has panacea-like properties, and before long, this is showing to be the circumstance. On August eleventh, 2013, Sanjay Gupta discharged a record on CNN about Charlotte Figi. Charlotte is a fiery Dravet issue quiet who was having 300 thousand mal seizures seven days. No pharmaceuticals or dietary changes could reasonably diminish this number. Charlotte's kin found a few solutions concerning high-CBD cannabis oil, and after extremely the fundamental piece, Charlotte's seizures halted. She right presently has under three minor seizures a month. This case is completely extraordinary, and it's not isolated. Dr. Margaret Gedde, a Colorado Springs pro, is following 11 new patients of the Stanely family, the suppliers of Charlotte's high-CBD medicine. 9 of them have had 90-100% reduces in seizures, which once more, is essentially superb.

The epileptic conditions that CBD is exhibiting to constrain against are inconceivably amazing, and for no situation the most predominant, all around investigated pharmaceuticals have been prepared for impelling any repairing. Anyway high-CBD cannabis oil is rapidly and seriously reducing reactions, with the fundamental indications being basically useful - greater imperativeness, better learning, improved lead, and that is just a hint of something larger.

It should not be astounding that results like these have been proceeding for an extensive period of time. Much equivalent to research shows cannabinoids are remedially feasible against epilepsy, there is research proposing they can crash threatening developments and control distinctive real illnesses. Additionally, before long, for epilepsy and these various conditions, the results are importance individuals. People have been reliably taking out tumors for an extensive period of time and directing contaminations as crohn diabetes, fibromyalgia, coronary disease, consistent torment, various sclerosis, and that is only the start. This is pretty much veritable; more thought must be brought to this issue essentialness and mental state.

CANNABIS OIL A CANCER TREATMENT ALTERNATIVE TO CHEMOTHERAPY?

The THS in cannabis oil connects to the CB2 and CB1 cannabinoid receptors inside of cancerous cells. This leads to an influx of ceramide synthesis, which causes cancer cells to die. The great thing about this is that unlike chemotherapy, cannabis oil only adversely affects cancer cells, not healthy cells. Normal cells don't produce ceramide when exposed to THC, which is why it goes untouched. The cytotoxic chemicals aren't what causes the cancer cells to die - it's the small shift in the mitochondria, which acts as the energy source for cell.

HOW CBD OIL HELPS IN APOPTOSIS

Apoptosis is a characteristic procedure in the body where the cells are decimated as a major aspect of a specific creature's development. As referenced, disease cells develop as an unusual procedure in the body since they never again recognize the body's flag that empower or decimate cell development. As these cells develop and partition, they become increasingly wild. What's more, since they never again react to apoptosis, they will in general speed up cell expansion and disregard different sign from typical cells? That is the reason the endocannabinoid framework is a critical framework in the body since it likewise helps in balancing cell development and demise. As disease cells duplicate quicker than the endocannabinoid framework can deal with, the malignancy cells attack through the typical tissues and spread all through the body. This procedure is called metastasis.

The endocannabinoid framework has two essential receptors. One is the CB1 receptors which are for the most part found in the mind, and the other one is the CB2 receptors which are fundamentally found in the invulnerable framework. THC is the dynamic compound in cannabis that ties to the CB1 receptors and is answerable for state of mind, conduct, and other cerebral capacities. Then again, CBD locks onto the CB2 receptors and tells these receptors if there are trespassers? that are inconvenient to the body. The apoptotic procedure by these receptors is accomplished through the all over again union of ceramide and sphingolipid that advance cell pulverization. When they tie together, the receptor enactment would then be able to help the endocannabinoid framework in flagging an antitumorigenic cautioning. This implies, it impedes malignancy advancement through hindering reproduction, metastasis, and tumor angiogenesis.

With the developing number of states, the nation over that have invited enactment making marijuana legitimate, both medically and recreationally, new products are in effect explicitly custom fitted to the maturing populace. One such product, which comes in numerous structures, is Cannabidiol or CBD. CBD which can be conveyed in numerous manners including oil fume, topical cream, ingestible tinctures or edibles, is the non-psychoactive part found in marijuana. In layman terms, CBD conveys the entirety of the advantages of marijuana without making the client high. The constructive outcomes that are expedited utilizing CBD can be especially inviting to seniors.

Numerous seniors don't know about how medical cannabis could improve their personal satisfaction and how the cliché marijuana client and use has changed. Since CBD is extricated from the marijuana plant, seniors can exploit the medical advantages managed by the concentrate without the head or body sensation regularly connected with marijuana. Moreover, seniors have the choice of conveying CBD to their bodies in structures increasingly recognizable, instead of breathing in smoke. CBD is an oil concentrate and consequently can be added to things like topical gels, tinctures and eatable products.

Much of the time, these subordinates of cannabis can lessen or even supplant the utilization of unsafe and addictive professionally prescribed drugs. While this data is just presently advancing into the standard, the characteristic outcome is, seniors drop their preferences, face reality and go to the treatment of their minor and noteworthy age-related diseases using cannabis.

Here are 8 reasons why CBD should turn into a customary piece of each senior's health normal as they age.

1. HELP WITH DISCOMFORT

It has for quite some time been realized that cannabis is a torment reliever to a similar degree as, maybe stunningly better, professionally prescribed medicine. For example, clinical investigations have demonstrated that Marijuana is exceptionally successful in diminishing joint pain and nerve torment. Carefully assembled, medical, boutique-style creams are the successful fix of various muscles and joint torments.

2. BONE HEALTH

CBD Oil Cannabis could give an extraordinary need to the older as it identifies with bone delicacy. As indicated by an examination, cannabis use can help mend cracks and bolster healthier bones. As a result of its calming properties, cannabis can be extremely valuable for patients with different sclerosis.

3. ALLEVIATING EFFECTS

In spite of the fact that CBD is known for its mitigating consequences for senior shoppers, it advances the sentiment of vitality and acts against latency. This is on the grounds that CBD reinforces cells in the human body and adds to finish recovery. What's more, CBD is a cell reinforcement that advances the feeling of carefulness that can be upset by the nearness of free radicals. A study shows that cannabidiol has more grounded cancer prevention agent properties than Vitamin C and Vitamin E.

4. BATTLES GLAUCOMA

There has been developing research that supports a connection among cannabis and the treatment of glaucoma. Glaucoma, which is a neurodegenerative malady (the breakdown of neurons in the correspondence procedure from the mind to the body), influences seeing people from an expansion in pressure in the eye known as intraocular pressure (IoP). Returning decades, there is supporting proof that cannabinoids can decrease IoP by up to 25%, anyway the necessary measurement of inward breath of full THC cannabis has represented a hazard to certain patients. Nonetheless, because of the going with manifestations of glaucoma, CBD as a torment the board product functions admirably, and may have the additional advantage of decreasing pressure.

5. A SLEEPING DISORDER AND SLEEP ISSUES

The more seasoned we get, the more troublesome it is to accomplish continued times of profound rest. During the profound rest stages, our mind recovers and is liberated from poisonous substances, which were delivered by the body itself. Along these lines, rest quality is additionally of colossal significance to avoid age-related neurodegenerative sicknesses, for example, Alzheimer's illness or glaucoma. Every now and again, older individuals are recommended resting pills, which have an incredible potential for reliance and a wide scope of horrendous symptoms. CBD can help in the augmentation of the profound rest stage and the decrease of the lighter dozing stages.

6. OPTION IN CONTRAST TO PRESCRIPTION MEDICATIONS

The quantity of seniors who utilize every day physician endorsed drugs develops every year pointlessly and persistently. Pharmaceutical organizations present our legislature with one of the biggest campaigning bunches in the nation, to advance the viability and dependability gave by their products. In any case, professionally prescribed drugs can be very perilous for its clients, and can be liable for organ harm, tissue harm, chronic drug use and even demise. In examination, marijuana is a protected option in contrast to physician endorsed drugs, accompanying less symptoms and lower addictive attributes. This advantage is increased with CBD and in reality, has been utilized to battle dependence on doctor prescribed drugs. Neither passings nor overdoses have been archived, which are identified with marijuana.

7. ANIMATES APPETITE

A general, risky health danger among more established residents is the loss of craving, which causes weight reduction, tissue shortcoming, and mental issues. While marijuana has been widely researched, and appeared to improve the hunger of clients, CBD in like manner has demonstrated to be a decent craving stimulant and along these lines supportive for seniors.

8. ALZHEIMER'S AND DEMENTIA

A developing pattern that is being researched is could marijuana forestall the beginning of Alzheimer's illness. As indicated by various investigations, cannabinoids, and by expansion CBD, can add to the end of a dangerous protein identified with this ailment. This is activated by lost aggravation of the mind and recovery of harmed cells.

USEFULNESS OF CANNABIS OIL FOR THE AGED

With the developing number of states, the nation over that have invited enactment making marijuana legitimate, both medically and recreationally, new products are as a rule explicitly customized to the maturing populace. One such product, which comes in numerous structures, is Cannabidiol or CBD. CBD which can be conveyed in numerous manners including oil fume, topical cream, ingestible tinctures or edibles, is the non-psychoactive part found in marijuana. In layman terms, CBD conveys the entirety of the advantages of marijuana without making the client high. The beneficial outcomes that are expedited utilizing CBD can be especially inviting to seniors. Numerous seniors don't know about how medical cannabis could improve their personal satisfaction and how the cliché marijuana client and use has changed. Since CBD is removed from the marijuana plant, seniors can exploit the medical advantages managed by the concentrate without the head or body sensation regularly connected with marijuana.

Moreover, seniors have the alternative of conveying CBD to their bodies in structures progressively commonplace, as opposed to breathing in smoke. CBD is an oil concentrate and, in this manner, can be added to things like topical gels, tinctures and eatable products. Much of the time, these subsidiaries of cannabis can lessen or even supplant the utilization of destructive and addictive professionally prescribed drugs. While this data is just currently advancing into the standard, the characteristic outcome is, seniors drop their partialities, face the truth and go to the treatment of their minor and significant age-related ailments utilizing cannabis.

Here are 8 reasons why CBD should turn into a normal part of each senior's health standard as they age.

1. RELIEF FROM DISCOMFORT

It has for some time been realized that cannabis is a torment reliever to a similar degree as, maybe shockingly better, physician recommended medicine. For example, clinical examinations have demonstrated that Marijuana is exceptionally viable in diminishing joint pain and nerve torment. High quality, medical, boutique-style creams are the powerful fix of various muscles and joint torments.

2. BONE HEALTH

CBD Oil Cannabis could give an incredible need to the older as it identifies with bone delicacy. As indicated by an examination, cannabis use can help mend breaks and bolster healthier bones. In view of its mitigating properties, cannabis can be exceptionally valuable for patients with various sclerosis.

3. MITIGATING EFFECTS

Despite the fact that CBD is known for its relieving consequences for senior purchasers, it advances the sentiment of vitality and acts against latency. This is on the grounds that CBD fortifies cells in the human body and adds to finish recovery. Also, CBD is a cell reinforcement that advances the feeling of carefulness that can be upset by the nearness of free radicals. A study shows that cannabidiol has more grounded cell reinforcement properties than Vitamin C and Vitamin E.

4. BATTLES GLAUCOMA

There has been developing research that supports a connection among cannabis and the treatment of glaucoma. Glaucoma, which is a neurodegenerative ailment (the breakdown of neurons in the correspondence procedure from the cerebrum to the body), influences seeing people from an expansion in pressure in the eye known as intraocular pressure (IoP). Returning decades, there is supporting proof that cannabinoids can diminish IoP by up to 25%, anyway the necessary measurement of inward breath of full THC cannabis has represented a hazard to certain patients. Be that as it may, because of the going with side effects of glaucoma, CBD as an agony the executive's product functions admirably, and may have the additional advantage of diminishing weight.

5. A SLEEPING DISORDER AND SLEEP ISSUES

The more seasoned we get, the more troublesome it is to accomplish supported times of profound rest. During the profound rest stages, our cerebrum recovers and is liberated from harmful substances, which were delivered by the body itself. Along these lines, rest quality is additionally vital to counteract age-related neurodegenerative sicknesses, for example, Alzheimer's illness or glaucoma. As often as possible, old individuals are recommended dozing pills, which have an extraordinary potential for reliance and a wide scope of upsetting reactions. CBD can help in the expansion of the profound rest stage and the decrease of the lighter dozing stages.

6. OPTION IN CONTRAST TO PRESCRIPTION MEDICATIONS

The quantity of seniors who utilize every day doctor prescribed drugs develops every year pointlessly and constantly. Pharmaceutical organizations present our legislature with one of the biggest campaigning bunches in the nation, to advance the adequacy and security gave by their products. Be that as it may, doctor prescribed drugs can be incredibly perilous for its clients, and can be liable for organ harm, tissue harm, chronic drug use and even demise. In correlation, marijuana is a protected option in contrast to physician recommended drugs, accompanying less symptoms and lower addictive attributes. This advantage is elevated with CBD and in truth has been utilized to battle dependence on physician endorsed drugs. Neither passing nor overdoses have been recorded, which are identified with marijuana.

7. ANIMATES APPETITE

A general, hazardous health danger among more established residents is the loss of craving, which causes weight reduction, tissue shortcoming, and mental issues. While marijuana has been broadly researched, and appeared to improve the hunger of clients, CBD in like manner has demonstrated to be a decent craving stimulant and consequently supportive for seniors.

8. ALZHEIMER'S AND DEMENTIA

A rising pattern that is being researched is could marijuana counteract the beginning of Alzheimer's malady. As indicated by various investigations, cannabinoids, and by expansion CBD, can add to the end of a harmful protein identified with this ailment. This is

98

activated by lost irritation of the cerebrum and recovery of damaged cells.

CANNABIS PHARMACY OIL ON PETS

HOW IS CBD CONTROLLED TO ANIMALS?

CBD pet consideration products come in a significant number of similar structures you're most likely used to seeing for people, including edibles (think: chewable treats and cases), oils that can be added to nourishment or set under the tongue and topical creams or emollients that are scoured legitimately on the skin. Like the CBD products implied for people, every one of these CBD pet care product types seems to differently affect the body - in dogs, in any case. When McGrath began examining CBD in 2016, one of her first examinations investigated how three diverse conveyance techniques - a container, an oil and a cream - influenced the way CBD traveled through the assortments of healthy dogs. "We quantified the pharmacokinetics, which fundamentally implies you give the dogs a solitary portion of every one of the three conveyance strategies and afterward you measure a lot of various blood levels over a 12-hour time frame," says McGrath. "So how rapidly is the CBD ingested, how high the blood fixation gets at that solitary portion, and afterward how quick the CBD is killed."

McGrath found that out of the three explicit plans they tried, the oil had the best pharmacokinetic profile, which means it arrived at the most elevated fixation in the blood, remained in the circulatory system the longest, and played out the most reliably over the various dogs. The case additionally performed well however the cream less so. It performed too conflictingly for McGrath and her group to reach any inferences. These outcomes line up with what we know so far about CBD assimilation in people, yet the research is too primer to be in any way used to settle on any medical choices.

In spite of the fact that there are some topical medications, cannabis oil is regularly managed orally to dogs. It additionally can be utilized related to customary medications and medicines. Rising research proposes there can be "synergistic benefits" among marijuana and conventional medications, Richter says. "There are scarcely any, known critical medication collaborations that you truly should be worried about." Again, the right measurement is basic. "Just like the case with any medication, achievement has an inseparable tie to dosing," Richter says. "In the event that you portion pets appropriately, at that point they will get the beneficial outcome that you're searching for while not having any psychoactive symptoms." But thus, lies an issue. The research expected to decide the right measurements for CBD oil in dogs essentially hasn't been done at this point, Coates says. Also, to exacerbate the situation, FDA testing has indicated that numerous CBD products contain pretty much nothing if any CBD, she includes. The best alternative accessible to pet guardians right now is to converse with a veterinarian who has involvement in pets being treated with cannabis oil about appropriate measurement and trustworthy makers, Coates says.

HOW DOES CBD WORK IN ANIMALS?

It's hazy - and a riddle researcher are as yet attempting to unravel in people too. For example, dogs have an endocannabinoid framework however whether CBD communicates with it similarly specialists figure it does in people is not yet clear. For the present, all McGrath knows is that in dogs, as in people, CBD seems, by all accounts, to be utilized by the liver.

ARE THERE ANY HEALTH ADVANTAGES TO GIVING YOUR PET CBD?

Once more, it's too soon to tell. A recent report found that CBD can assist increment with encouraging and action in dogs with osteoarthritis and the next year McGrath distributed an examination demonstrating CBD may help lessen the quantity of seizures experienced by epileptic dogs. In any case, despite the fact that these examinations were well-planned and peer-evaluated, they're still little and extremely starter. "All we've essentially done is give this medication to these dogs and stated, OK, this is what we're seeing," says McGrath. "Yet, regardless of whether the blood levels accomplished are sufficient enough to treat certain ailments, we don't yet have the foggiest idea." Still, McGrath is hopeful. Veterinarians don't have a wide assortment of drugs accessible to treat these conditions and a portion of the ones that do exist regularly accompany weakening reactions, for example, weight increase and laziness. "On the off chance that CBD works, at that point I figure it would hit the sign of being both successful and not conveying a ton of symptoms," says McGrath. "So's sort of what we're seeking after."

McGrath and different researchers across the country are at present leading bigger investigations on CBD's adequacy in treating osteoarthritis in dogs and cats, epilepsy in dogs and post-employable torment, yet it will be some time before the outcomes are distributed. Until more is known, it's ideal to converse with your veterinarian before giving your creature CBD.

CBD, in its unadulterated state, radiates an impression of being ensured and well-suffered by animals, as showed by a 2017 World Health Organization report. Regardless, both resulting 2018 canine examinations referenced above saw an extension in the liver substance solvent phosphatase (ALP) during CBD treatment. As a segment of her assessment, McGrath ran a simultaneous liver limit test to guarantee the dogs' livers weren't missing the mark and everything returned commonplace so it's dim whether the raised ALP levels were achieved by something absolutely positive or could shape into a continuously significant issue whole deal. "I would be a little stressed over offering CBD to a canine that has known liver issues," says McGrath. Furthermore, because CBD has every one of the reserves of being prepared by the liver, McGrath says she'd similarly be careful about offering CBD to a canine who starting at now takes a solution that is used by the liver. "We don't by and large have the foggiest thought regarding these things interface right now," she says. The different colossal thing pet owners should think about is quality control. Since the CBD market isn't especially overseen now, CBD products can contain fixings that aren't recorded on their names - including THC, which is known to be hazardous to cats and dogs.

One way to deal with avoid perhaps hazardous fixings is to simply use products that go with a confirmation of assessment, or COA (the cluster number on the COA should arrange the number on the product's name or packaging). A COA is given when a self-sufficient lab tests the product to assert its fixings and quality, notwithstanding different things. Genuinely, CBD products must contain near 0.3% THC, which should be okay for animals. Nonetheless, there's no inspiration to go for broke. At whatever point possible, stick to CBD pet thought products that contain 0.0% THC and be attentive for signs of THC hurting, for instance, spewing, detachment of the entrails, torpidity, tension and issue standing. Essential concern: "We haven't found whatever's excessively upsetting about CBD," says McGrath. "However, on the opposite side, in spite of all that we know beside no about it and it's very critical for owners to understand that and use it with alert until we have more information."

WHAT ARE THE BENEFITS OF CANNABIS OIL FOR DOGS?

Cannabis oil can be used to treat seizures, ailment, stress, pressure, joint aggravation, back desolation, appearances of dangerous development, and gastrointestinal issues, among other wellbeing conditions in dogs. Help is given as the cannabinoids in marijuana work together with the endocannabinoid system, Shu explains. "It's a movement of receptors that run all through the body," he says. "The cannabinoids team up with the receptors in the body and direct things like torment, uneasiness, and nausea." Unlike some ordinary torment medicine for dogs, medical cannabis has no unsafe responses with authentic portion, Shu points out. "It doesn't hurt the kidney, liver, or GI tract. The dogs aren't high or quieted."

WHAT ARE THE POTENTIAL RISKS OF CANNABIS OIL FOR PETS?

Like any meds, overdosing can incite potential dangers for pets. "The hugest is THC dangerous quality, which infers, basically, they are high," Richter says. "Subordinate upon how unmitigated a pet has been overdosed, the impacts of that can be amazingly enduring, even days." During these scenes, a pet will no doubt be not capable stand or eat. On the off chance that you accept an overdose, take your pet to the veterinarian right away. Dangerous dangers for dogs from medical cannabis are "exceedingly striking," Richter says, including that lethality much more periodically happens when a pet has eaten a product that contains chocolate, espresso, or raisins. "In spite of whether the THC harmful quality isn't outrageous, they can a segment of the time have issues because of these different fixings." That communicated, ingestion of a huge amount of marijuana has been fatal in various dogs, so defeating overdoses with medical cannabis is so far fundamental, cautions Dr. Jennifer Coates, a veterinary expert with petMD.

Graham Quigley, proprietor and acupuncturist at the Holistic Animal Clinic in San Rafael, California, centers around that as the normality of elective medicine amasses, pet guards may get tied up with "irrationally aching cases about cannabis oil" from defective sources. Quigley stresses that cannabis oil isn't a "fix all." As with any medicine, pet guards should coordinate their veterinarian first before treating their canine with cannabis oil.

WHERE CAN PET OWNERS GET CANNABIS OIL FOR THEIR DOGS?

Getting medical cannabis for your pet all depends upon where you live and your state's marijuana laws. "In California, to legitimately buy marijuana, you should have a medical cannabis card, which an individual would get from their primary care physician," Richter says. "There is no lawful system by which I, as a veterinarian, can give a medical cannabis card to a pet." Pet owners who need to give their pooch cannabis oil should address their veterinarian. From that point, pet guardians who have a medical marijuana card can visit a legitimate dispensary and buy the product that best addresses their pet's issues. Pet guardians who live in areas where medical marijuana isn't accessible can likewise think about hemp products, which have lower portions of THC.

NEGATIVE IMPLICATIONS OF CANNABIS ABUSE ON GENERAL AND ORAL HEALTH

Cannabis, normally known as Marijuana, is the most as often as possible utilized unlawful medication in America. As indicated by National Survey on Drug Use and Health (NSDUH), there were about 15.2 million past month clients in America in 2008. It additionally expressed that about 2.2 million individuals utilized Marijuana without precedent for 2008.

These midpoints to around 6,000 Marijuana start for each day. Numerous individuals are getting dependent on Marijuana, unmindful of its destructive consequences for health. Today, Cannabis abuse is a huge worry because of its negative effects on general physical, mental and oral wellbeing.

There are three principle types of Cannabis: Marijuana, Hash and Hash oil, all of which contain the fundamental psychoactive constituent, 'Delta-9-Tetrahydrocannabinol', just called as THC. Cannabis misuse influences pretty much every arrangement of the body including the cardiovascular, respiratory, mental and oral frameworks.

A portion of the negative ramifications of Cannabis misuse are:

At the point when somebody smokes or devours Cannabis, THC goes from the lungs or stomach into the circulation system, which conveys the substance to the cerebrum and different organs all through the body. As indicated by National Institute on Drug Abuse (NIDA), pulse is expanded by 20 to 100 percent not long after smoking Marijuana.

It is additionally evaluated that Marijuana clients have very nearly multiple times danger of coronary episode in the principal hour in the wake of smoking Marijuana. Maturing individuals or those with heart vulnerabilities will be at higher hazard. Long haul smoking of Marijuana is related with negative impacts on the respiratory framework. The smoke from a Cannabis cigarette has indistinguishable substance from tobacco smoke separated from unsafe substance like carbon monoxide, bronchial aggravations, tar and more significant levels of different cancer-causing agents than in tobacco smoke. Constant smokers of Cannabis have expanded side effects of bronchitis, including hacking, wheezing, mucus production, increasingly visit intense chest ailment, and expanded danger of lung diseases.

The manifestations of bronchitis are more typical in Cannabis smokers than non-smokers of the medication. Cannabis misuse results in dysregulated development of epithelial cells in lungs, which may prompt malignancy.

CONSEQUENCES FOR MENTAL HEALTH

Intense impacts of Cannabis misuse fluctuate extraordinarily between people contingent upon the measurements, technique for organization, condition and character of the client. Long haul Cannabis misuse expands the danger of genuine mental diseases. THC follows up on explicit locales in the mind, called cannabinoid receptors. The most noteworthy thickness of cannabinoid receptors is found in parts of the cerebrum that impact joy, memory, musings, focus, tangible and time discernment and so forth. Clearly, Marijuana inebriation can cause misshaped recognitions, debilitated coordination, trouble in intuition and critical thinking, and issues with learning and memory. Marijuana misuse can expand paces of uneasiness, despondency, self-destructive ideation, and schizophrenia.

EFFECTS ON ORAL HEALTH

Cannabis clients are inclined to oral diseases. By and large, Cannabis abusers have more unfortunate oral health than non-clients, with higher rotted, absent and filled (DMF) teeth scores, higher plaque scores and less healthy teeth gums. A significant reaction of Cannabis misuse is xerostomia (dryness of the mouth brought about by failing salivary organs). Cannabis smoking and biting causes changes in the oral epithelium, named 'cannabis stomatitis'. Its side effects incorporate aggravation and shallow anesthesia of the oral membranous tissue covering inner organs. With ceaseless use, this may advance to neoplasia (development of a tumor).

CANNABIS USE CAUSES ORAL MALIGNANT GROWTH

Constant smokers of Cannabis have an expanded danger of creating oral leukoplakia (thick white fixes on mucous films of the oral cavity, including the tongue. It frequently happens as a pre-malignant development), oral disease and other oral contaminations. Oral malignancy identified with cannabis as a rule happens on the foremost floor of the mouth and the tongue. Cannabis utilization additionally has its effects on driving, influencing engine abilities, reflexes, and consideration. This builds coincidental dangers. Cannabis misuse can possibly mess up day by day life too. Cannabis misuse disables a few significant proportions of life accomplishment including physical and mental health, psychological capacities, public activity and profession status. The expanding commonness of Cannabis use requests familiarity with the different unfavorable effects of Cannabis misuse. Individuals should think about these effects and make auspicious move so as to avoid its negative ramifications.

RELATED EFFECTS ON USAGE OF CANNABIS PHARMACY OIL

Late studies have uncovered many of its advantages and introduced proof of its potential as a lot more secure alternative over numerous pharmaceutical drugs. Notwithstanding, there is still a great deal to be wanted as far research on this non-psychoactive cannabinoid is concerned. Because of the absence of broad investigation on its symptoms, it is frequently not exhorted by specialists even in places where medical marijuana is legitimate. Despite its advantages, this home grown concentrate, such as everything else we can ingest or use on ourselves, has certain symptoms. To comprehend the suitability of this medication as a potential solution for various illnesses, it is basic for us to think about CBD oil's reactions in some detail.

Unexpectedly, no instances of danger or overdose from utilization of hemp-based (modern evaluation hemp) CBD oil have been accounted for up until now. Actually, this specific concentrate of marijuana or hemp has been seen as very safe for use by nearly everybody. Dosages of up to 1500 mg of CBD have been believed to be effectively endured by human. Portions of up to 1500 mg of CBD have been believed to be effectively endured by human guineas pigs. CBD scarcely has any negative effect on people, may happen just in uncommon cases and that too in a gentle manner.

Be that as it may, there are connected effects on the use of CBD oil which are examined underneath;

- **Mouth Dryness:** This is a typical wonder among individuals who use CBD or some other cannabinoids, in the two instances of expending or smoking. A wonder, which feels like your mouth is loaded down with cotton balls, can be effectively overwhelmed by drinking a great deal of water or other hydrating liquids previously, during or after utilization of CBD. The explanation behind this is the point at which an individual devours or smokes any cannabinoid, the endocannabinoid framework, which has its receptors present in the salivary organs, represses the discharge of the organs. Ongoing considers (1) have found that the submandibular organ that produces over 60% of the spit has cannabinoid receptors. Anandamide,an endocannabinoid that causes dryness of mouth, interfaces with these receptors and hinders salivation production by obstructing the sign from the sensory system to create spit.

- **Sluggishness:** CBD oil regularly doesn't incite any sentiments of languor. Be that as it may, CBD's impact on people varies from individual to individual. As a rule, CBD has a wake-inciting impact, making an individual progressively alert and enthusiastic, while in others it can create the exact inverse response. In extremely high portions, the last classification of individuals has detailed inclination lazy in the wake of expending CBD. Diminishing the measurement can be a decent alternative. On the off chance that you have a place with this class of individuals, it is best for you to NOT work any substantial hardware or drive a vehicle, for your very own wellbeing and people around you. As another safety measure for individuals who experience sluggishness because of devouring CBD oil, lessening the dose can be a decent alternative.

- **Dazedness or Lightheadedness**: some tea or espresso can do some amazing things in such circumstances. A truly uncommon and impermanent reaction, unsteadiness can be effectively overseen by drinking a stimulated refreshment that will help your body rapidly recapture its typical equalization. Some tea or espresso can do some amazing things in such circumstances, yet try to drink a great deal of water alongside it, as caffeine has a drying out impact on the body.

- **Drop in Blood Pressure**: This is normally the motivation behind why a few people experience wooziness. While there is proof of CBD oil helping individuals with heart sicknesses and diabetes by bringing down their pulse, this nature of this cannabinoid can have negative effect on individuals with ordinary circulatory strain. As indicated by certain investigations, higher portions of CBD can cause a slight drop in pulse. Any product containing over 0.3% THC is Illegal. Along these lines, individuals who experience the ill effects of low circulatory strain or are taking medicine for it should cease from devouring CBD or CBD-based products. While it is in every case best to counsel a specialist before considering CBD oil as an elective treatment, whenever looked with such a circumstance, drinking espresso typically helps, much the same as if there should be an occurrence of wooziness.

- **Diarrhea and Change in Appetite and Weight:** In 2017, a clinical investigation of patients with epilepsy and insane issue and their response to CBD oil as a type of treatment was distributed in the diary, Cannabis and Cannabinoid Research. Over the span of their research, researchers found that the subjects encountered some regular symptoms like tiredness, loose bowels, and changes in both weight as well as hunger. Be that as it may, it was reasoned that: "In examination with different drugs, utilized for the treatment of these medical conditions, CBD has a superior reaction profile. "This study, in any case, left space for progressively broad research into the "toxicological parameters" of CBD oil, for occasion, its impact on hormones.

- **Impact on Patients with Movement Disorders**: A couple of increasingly potential threats of CBD use do even now exist, especially among patients of some prior conditions, for instance, among patients of dystonic development issue. Patients when treated with oral dosages of 100–600mg CBD oil every day. In an investigation, distributed in the International Journal of Neuroscience in 2009, such patients when treated with oral portions of 100–600mg CBD oil every day for a time of about a month and a half, close by standard prescriptions, gave indications of progress. In any case, that was likewise joined by the regular symptoms referenced above (low circulatory strain, dryness of mouth, languor and wooziness), alongside not really basic psychomotor easing back (or backing off of point of view and of physical developments). At the point when the portion was over 300 mg/day, symptoms like increment in hypokinesia and resting tremor were seen, uncovering one of the threats of utilizing CBD oil on patients of Parkinson's Disease. However, another examination, distributed in the Journal of Psychopharmacology recommended that utilization of CBD really improves the personal satisfaction in patients with Parkinson's disease. This goes to demonstrate that a great deal of research should be done around there to determine at an authoritative end in regards to the advantage as well as negative effect on patients of Parkinson's Disease.

INTERACTION WITH PHARMACEUTICAL DRUGS

Individuals taking any pharmaceutical prescription for a previous affliction or condition must be especially cautious about CBD's effects on medicate digestion inside the liver. CBD has been found to obstruct the movement of specific chemicals found in the liver –, for example, the cytochrome P450 compound framework (especially CYP3A4) – that processes pharmaceutical drugs implied for human utilization. P450 chemical framework contains in excess of 50 compounds. As indicated by Davis' Drug Guide, the P450 chemical framework contains in excess of 50 proteins that procedure and dispose of poisons. (7) If taken in high dosages, CBD oil can totally kill P450 protein's movement, as this cannabinoid requires a similar chemical to be processed. In addition, certain pharmaceutical drugs additionally restrain this protein. This mean the breakdown of CBD oil may get upset prompting an expansion in its physiological action.

Besides, there are sure pharmaceutical prescriptions that can really expand the degree of this chemical, bringing about quicker breakdown of CBD. Albeit such impedances may just be a minor and generally a brief issue, it is constantly protected to counsel your primary care physician before utilizing CBD oil alongside pharmaceutical drugs.

REACTIONS OF FDA-APPROVED DRUG FOR EPILEPSY

The US Food and Drug Administration endorsed Epidiolex (a CBD-based medication) oral answer for treatment of two kinds of epilepsy, Lennox-Gastaut Syndrome and Dravet Syndrome for patients matured 2 years or more. Be that as it may, throughout its clinical preliminaries, researchers found certain unfavorable effects (6) of the medication:

- Liver issues

- Manifestations identified with the focal sensory system like peevishness and torpidity

- Diminished hunger

- Gastrointestinal issues

- Diseases

- Rashes and other affectability responses

- Diminished pee

- Breathing issues

- Danger of intensifying emotional episodes, wretchedness or self-destructive propensities.

CBD (as talked about prior) restrains the breakdown of certain pharmaceutical drugs and, now and again, the other way around. This may prompt the nearness of more significant levels of these drugs in your framework, causing undesirable symptoms, now and then even an overdose. It is basic to take note of that CBD oil isn't the only one in this impact on medicate digestion. Grapefruit, watercress, St John's Wort, and goldenseal likewise hinder movement of the cytochrome P450 or CYP450. The drugs being referred to, any medication that requires the liver's CYP450 chemicals to utilize might associate with CBD oil. As indicated by the Indiana University Department of Medicine, drugs known to utilize the CYP450 framework incorporate (7):

- Steroids

- HMG CoA reductase inhibitors

- Calcium channel blockers

- Antihistamines

- Prokinetics

- HIV antivirals

- Insusceptible modulators

- Benzodiazepines

- Antiarrythmics

- Anti-infection agents

- Sedatives

- Antipsychotics

- Antidepressants

- Enemies of epileptics

- Beta blockers

- PPIs

- NSAIDs

- Angiotension II blockers

- Oral hypoglycemic specialists

- Sulfonylureas

It must be referenced here that this rundown isn't thorough and neither would it be able to be said with vindication that every one of these drugs will unfavorably respond with cannabidiol. It is best for you to counsel a medical expert before enhancing your treatment with CBD oil.

PRODRUG

There is additionally a gathering of medicines that fall under the "prodrug" classification. These are meds that should be used to the restorative compound. In other words, when you ingest an inert compound, it enters your framework and is then prepared into a functioning medication. In the event that this handling requires CYP3A4 (some portion of the bigger CYP450 framework), at that point CBD can hinder the response, leaving too minimal dynamic medication in the body for the ideal effect. Case in point: Codeine that is processed into morphine. Vyvanse and Concerta are two other pharmaceutical meds, implied for ADHD, which likewise fall under this classification.

WELLBEING CONCERNS

Cannabis is getting very well known as a protected and characteristic medicine, with for all intents and purposes zero lethality. Research has appraised this cannabinoid as least hazardous substance, when contrasted with substances, for example, liquor and nicotine concerning toxicity. But the inquiry is: Is CBD a characteristic nourishment supplement or a medicine? Most talks identifying with its lawful status relies upon that, since "restorative drugs are viewed as risky until demonstrated safe" while it is the polar opposite if there should arise an occurrence of characteristic supplements. Additionally, CBD oil is as yet unregulated, which means its right measurement is as yet obscure. Be that as it may, human examinations have demonstrated that CBD is very all around endured even up to a day by day portion of 1,500 mg. Cannabidiol is nearly sheltered when expended in proper dosages among grown-ups. CBD portions of up to 300 mg day by day have been utilized securely for as long as a half year. portions of 1200-1500 mg day by day have been utilized securely for as long as about a month. Cannabidiol under-the-tongue showers have been utilized in portions of 2.5 mg for as long as about fourteen days.

Believe it or not, as demonstrated by a progressing World Health Organization (WHO) review, "until this point in time, there is no evidence of recreational use of CBD or any broad wellbeing related issues related with the use of unadulterated CBD". While the unadulterated type of

CBD might be of a lot of advantage to mankind, the fundamental concern is the synthesis of the products that are being made accessible in the market. Here, we are discussing the nearness of Tetrahydrocannabinol (or THC) (instances of mislabeling) and contaminants.

Mislabeling: According to research paper distributed in the Journal of the American Medical Association in 2017, practically 70% of all CBD products sold online are mislabeled. This implies they could contain higher hints of THC (just 0.3% and lower is allowed in modern evaluation CBD or hemp oil) that could genuinely hurt patients with tension issue and other maniacal issue. Contaminants: Studies have uncovered that cannabis plants from uncontrolled sources might be polluted with different destructive substances that could prompt serious health risks. Contaminants that are for the most part included by makers incorporate synthetic concoctions added purposefully to increase its yield, weight, or power:

- Pesticides

- Metal particles

- Engineered cannabinoids (Fake pot) (15)

- Certain different components that may enter the plant accidentally are:

- Overwhelming metals

- Molds and microscopic organisms

- Aflatoxins

A valid example: An ongoing paper from the Netherlands Ministry of Environment and Health uncovered that more than 90 percent of the Dutch cannabis sold in cafés contains hints of unlawful yield security Items such as pesticides.

(16) Another case: pesticides are also found in cannabis sold under state law in California

[17] As well as in regenerative cannabis from licensed producers in Canada.

[18] The uplifting news is that most contaminants are very simple to recognize, on account of the presence of the numerous expert logical labs that routinely screen for such contaminants in nourishment crops, imported therapeutic plants or eatable oils. Similar lab techniques can be applied to test for contaminants in CBD oils.

WHEN SHOULD YOU AVOID CBD OIL?

While CBD oil has numerous restorative effects on the human body and psyche, there are times and circumstances when you ought to avoid CBD oil utilization or use.

DURING PREGNANCY

There is proof of the sick effects of marijuana products on babies, if the mother is utilizing it during her pregnancy or while she is as yet breastfeeding her youngster (20, 21 and 22). Be that as it may, there is no such proof with respect to CBD in its unaltered structure, which has only 0.3 per cent THC and no more. As indicated by certain researchers, since cannabinoid receptors are engaged with mental health, CBD oil may upset fetal mental health. In any case, others are of the sentiment that CBD may, truth be told, advance healthy fetal mental health, since CBD can advance neurogenesis.

AWFUL FOR CHILDREN BENEATH 2 YEARS OF AGE

Without legitimate guidelines and adequate watchfulness over the closeout of CBD products, it isn't protected to oversee CBD in any structure to infants and kids underneath the age of 2 years. What impact even the small hints of THC may have on your infant and whether your child may get influenced by the following components of contaminants are not dangers you'd need to take with your little one's health. It is ideal to guarantee you are utilizing CBD in its most perfect structure and that too simply in the wake of counseling a specialist experienced in CBD's effects.

WHEN TAKING ANTIPSYCHOTIC, ANTIDEPRESSANT DRUGS

This has been clarified before in "What are the drugs that CBD connects with?" and a sub-segment under "Are there any reactions to utilizing CBD oil?"

OUTLINE

Despite its security concerns, it is verifiable how many individuals are progressively picking CBD products over pharmaceutical ones for the treatment of various illnesses – both physical and mental. This is generally because of its fewer reactions and by nil possibility of overdosing. Exploiting the ascent popular, a lot of corrupt makers and cannabis cultivators have come into the business with the sole expectation of profiting, without paying a lot of thought to the welfare of the individuals to whom they sell their products. In line with this, it is up to us as buyers to be careful and to do our own research before we take the risk of CBD products accessible on the market, in particular online ones.

IS ALL CANNABIS OIL THE SAME?

Before getting into the particular advantages of cannabis oil, it's critical to comprehend the various kinds of cannabis oil that are available. Cannabis and hemp plants contain diverse cannabinoids. These are substance parts that have some impact on you when expended. The two most regular cannabinoids are THC and CBD. Many tinctures, oils and cannabis products currently contain a certain proportion of THC and CBD. THC is the one that has brought the "high" to the vast majority of marijuana partners. Once, CBD is commonly used for restorative purposes.

The principle sorts of cannabis oil include:

CBD oil. This is a nonpsychoactive cannabis product. It doesn't contain THC, so it won't deliver a "high." CBD oil is prized for its restorative effects, including facilitating uneasiness, agony, and symptoms of chemotherapy.

Hemp-determined oil. Hemp is fundamentally the same as the cannabis plant, however it doesn't have any THC. It can contain CBD, yet its quality is typically viewed as the second rate. All things considered; hemp-determined oil can be a decent choice on the off chance that you live in a territory that hasn't legitimized cannabis.

Marijuana-inferred oil. Cannabis oil separated from a similar plant as dried marijuana leaves and buds has a higher proportion of THC. Subsequently, it has psychoactive effects.

Rick Simpson Oil (Rso). RSO contains elevated levels of THC with next to zero CBD. When picking a cannabis oil, make a point to deliberately take a gander at the name so you comprehend what proportion of THC to CBD you're getting.

HEMP OIL VERSUS CBD OIL

Most strikingly, the various terms to portray hemp, CBD and the different hemp-inferred products are particularly confounding. Huge numbers of the words are utilized reciprocally, however can mean altogether different things.

Is it hemp oil? CBD oil? Hemp seed oil? Shouldn't something be said about Hemp CBD to extricate? At that point there's cannabis oil, marijuana remove, the rundown continues forever.

Numerous enormous purchaser brands are likewise hopping onto the CBD temporary fad from CVS to Ben and Jerry's Ice Cream to Coca Cola. While these are unquestionably energizing occasions for the business, it's critical to comprehend the wording and truly realize what you're obtaining. The expression "hemp oil" may allude to either hemp seed oil or CBD oil, however CBD oil ought to never be utilized to portray hemp seed oil, I know, confounding!

While both hemp seed oil and CBD oil share certain attributes, and both have their advantages, there are some significant contrasts. In this book, we will concentrate on the contrasts between hemp seed oil and CBD Oil.

So, first of all, how do we characterize a few terms:

Cannabis:

Cannabis is a plant in the family Cannabaceae, beginning from Central Asia. There are three fundamental types of cannabis:

- Cannabis Indica

- Cannabis Sativa

- Cannabis Ruderalis

MARIJUANA

Marijuana is an assortment of cannabis sativa that contains a high measure of THC, which is the concoction (cannabinoid) liable for its inebriating effects. Marijuana is utilized for both medical or potentially recreational purposes. On account of marijuana's high THC content and psychoactive properties, it has been esteemed unlawful in numerous pieces of the world, including the US. Despite the fact that an ever-increasing number of states are sanctioning recreational marijuana as of late, it stays delegated a Schedule 1 medication on a government level.

HEMP

Like marijuana, hemp is another assortment of cannabis sativa, however has a much lower convergence of THC (0.3% or less). Hemp is broadly collected for modern uses, for example, paper, development materials and materials. In light of the low measure of THC, hemp has likewise been developed for non-tranquilize use as a health supplement.

CBD

CBD represents Cannabidiol. CBD is a concoction compound found in cannabis and has numerous therapeutic advantages, for example, calming and hostile to nervousness properties with no psychoactive effects.

CBD is available in all cannabis strains, including both marijuana and hemp assortments.

Note: CBD got from marijuana is as yet illicit in the US because of the high THC content in marijuana. Hemp-determined CBD is governmentally legitimate in the US under the 2018 Farm Bill since hemp contains under 0.3% THC. In this way, the lawfulness of CBD lies in the key expression "got from hemp".

What Is Hemp Seed Oil?

Hemp seed oil, which is here and there alluded to as hemp oil, is extricated by cool squeezing the seeds of the hemp plant. This is like how olive oil or coconut oil is sourced. The hemp seed oil has been accessible in health nourishment stores for quite a long time. It very well may be found in products, for example, cooking oil, moisturizers, skin care, beauty care products and cleansers.

What's the value of Hemp Seed Oil?

Hemp seed oil is known as a superfood because it contains high levels of cancer prevention agents, vitamins, minerals and amino acids. Hemp seeds contain huge measures of omega-3 and - 6 unsaturated fats, which can help decrease the indications of maturing, improve cardiovascular health and add to bring down the cholesterol levels. Hemp seeds are an extraordinary plant-based wellspring of protein, which makes hemp seed oil an ideal wellspring of complete protein for veggie lovers and vegetarians. Hemp seed oil is additionally an incredible lotion, and can be utilized to help hydrate your hair, nails and skin without stopping up your pores.

As a result of hemp seed's numerous health and nourishing advantages, everybody could utilize somewhat more hemp seed oil in their lives. The main downside of the hemp seed oil is that it doesn't contain any cannabinoids (THC, CBD, and so on), terpenes or other therapeutic mixes found in the stalks, leaves and blooms of the cannabis plant. This implies it doesn't furnish any of the advantages related to entire plant hemp separates.

What is CBD Oil?

CBD oil is gotten from the stalks, leaves and blooms ("airborne parts") of the cannabis plant. Since the hemp strain of cannabis contains low degrees of THC, CBD got from hemp won't make you "high". The proportion of high CBD to low THC makes hemp plants perfect for making CBD oil (and lawful!). CBD oil is removed from hemp utilizing either ethanol or CO2 extraction process... more on that later. There are various kinds of CBD oil extricated from hemp including full range, expansive range and CBD confine. For a point by point clarification about the upsides and downsides of each, read our past post here. CBD oil can once in a while be alluded to as CBD extricate, hemp removes or phytocannabinoid-rich (PCR) hemp separate.

What are the Benefits of CBD oil?

CBD oil got from hemp works with the body through the endocannabinoid framework (ECS). The endocannabinoid framework is liable for advancing homeostasis, which is the body's capacity to keep up parity and capacity appropriately. The ECS is ensnared is managing a significant number of our body's capacities, for example, rest, state of mind, torment, craving, hormone, and resistant reaction.

Taking CBD oil can help with an assortment of health-related issues, for example,

- Nervousness and sadness

- Relief from discomfort

- Hostile to aggravation

- Rest conditions

- Neurological issue

- Substance misuse

- Intellectual capacities

- Significance of Knowing the Difference

Run a quest on Amazon for CBD oil and you'll discover plenty of "Hemp Oil" products, yet what does that really mean? Clue: it's presumably not what you think. In the event that you unwittingly buy hemp seed oil thinking you'll receive the rewards of CBD; you will be significantly frustrated. Likewise, removing CBD oil is a substantially more muddled procedure than cold squeezing hemp seeds, along these lines CBD oil products are significantly more costly contrasted with hemp seed oil. A few advertisers are attempting to get on board with the CBD temporary fad and advancing hemp seed oil in a similar way as CBD, fooling purchasers into paying a premium for regular hemp seed oil. On the off chance that you fall prey to this strategy, your wallet will likewise be enormously frustrated. It's likewise critical to comprehend what to search for when purchasing CBD products. Unfortunately, most companies falsely say that their drug gives CBD, when it does not contain any.

WHAT TO LOOK FOR WHEN YOU BUY CBD OIL

Hemp seed oil is generally straight forward as far as naming is concerned. It's an alternative story for CBD products. Using your new phrase learning will significantly allow you to decode what you need to look for when assessing CBD oil products. If you're interested in trying CBD just because, start by reading our Beginner's CBD Guide. *Here are some extra tips:*

1. Ensure you read the marks to guarantee that CBD, Cannabidiol or "Phytocannabinoid-rich (PCR) hemp" is recorded as fixing just as the sum recorded, regularly in milligrams.

2. Ensure you know whether the product contains any THC. A few people will most likely be unable to ingest THC because of lawful purposes, breezing through a medication test, or some other individual reasons.

3. Ask what extraction strategy is utilized to remove CBD from hemp. Indication: CO_2 extraction is free of unsafe solvents and utilizations a delicate, low temperature, liquor free extraction process that yields the most flawless type of CBD Oil.

4. Read through COA's (Certificate of Analysis) and lab test results to guarantee they can back up their cases.

5. Find out about the organization, its notoriety and their arrival approach. Ensure they can address any inquiries or concerns you have about their products.

6. Peruse online audits for the products you're considering to check whether others have encountered positive outcomes.

Key Takeaways

- Marijuana and hemp are two unique strains of the cannabis plant.

- Hemp seed oil originates from hemp, while CBD oil can be obtained from either marijuana or hemp.

- Hemp seed oil and CBD oil have both their advantages, although there are significant differences between them. Hemp seed oil is separated by chilly squeezing hemp seeds, while CBD oil is extricated from the stalks, leaves and blooms of the plant.

- "Hemp oil" may allude to either hemp seed oil or CBD oil.

Medication testing has gotten normal in numerous working environments, and obligatory for those in government positions, law authorization, avionics, health and crisis medical consideration, and sports (especially those tried for prohibited substances). What numerous CBD clients don't understand is that follow measures of THC (the psychoactive compound in cannabis) can be found in CBD products, representing a potential danger of a positive medication test. All in all, what do you do in case your medication tried in your calling, yet need to encounter the health advantages of CBD? You can either avoid the substance through and through or you can take a safe CBD elective that takes a shot at your endocannabinoid framework superior to CBD alone.

How the Endocannabinoid System Works

To start with, it's critical to comprehend the endocannabinoid framework or ECS. You might be acquainted with this generally new term yet at the same time confounded about what it is actually. The endocannabinoid framework is 600-million-years of age, yet as of late found in the late '80s by a researcher researching the cannabis plant. What researchers found was a complex and wise body-wide receptor site framework that is responsible for managing rest wake cycles, temperament, tension and stress, digestion, vitality, agony and irritation, mental health, and much more.

While it has nothing to do with getting "high," the ECS is an unbelievably significant framework that has a vital influence in the guideline, upkeep, and parity of ideal health and recuperating. "The ECS with its activities in our resistant framework, sensory system, and all the body's organs, is truly a scaffold among body and brain," says Dustin Sulak, DO.

How CBD Affects the Body

Since you discover somewhat more about how the ECS functions, we should plunge into how CBD collaborates with this framework and influences the body. Your endocannabinoid framework requires "activators" called cannabinoids. Some cannabinoids are created normally in your body, called endocannabinoids and others are gotten from plants (like hemp or cannabis) called phytocannabinoids. These cannabinoids tie to receptor locales (CB1 and CB2) like a key does to a lock and may discharge a perplexing course of synapses that impart essential data to cells, tissues, organs, and organs basic to keeping up ideal health and homeostasis. In any case, researchers have found many non-cannabis and non-hemp plants that additionally contain mending phytocannabinoids that can initiate and support the endocannabinoid framework. This implies you can accomplish similar outcomes with different alternatives.

Did you say Non-Cannabis Cannabinoids?

Truly, believe it or not. Furthermore, you may as of now be acquainted with a portion of these non-cannabis plants, for example, ginger, echinacea and clove oil. Non-cannabis plants can imitate the movement of
130

cannabinoids yet have an alternate structure called cannabimimetic mixes and might be more successful at enacting the endocannabinoid framework than CBD alone. This is particularly incredible news for people who can't take CBD or who need to avoid the shame of cannabis and hemp.

All in all, what are the names of these non-cannabis cannabinoids?

Here's a short rundown of probably the most dominant herbs and botanicals containing phytocannabinoids that can assume a key job in your health.

Ginger root: One of the most powerful mitigating plants, ginger root is wealthy in the two cell reinforcements and cannabinoids. Since irritation can significantly affect your tissues, muscles, and joints, ginger root is basic to incorporate into your eating regimen. It normally supports the ECS by connecting to receptors liable for managing agony and aggravation.

- **Magnolia:** Experts have found that magnolia bark and its fundamental bioactive mixes (magnolol and honokiol) have calming, hostile to bacterial and against unfavorably susceptible specialists. Moreover, magnolia can initiate cannabinoid receptors answerable for controlling rest, memory, and uneasiness.

- **Dark pepper:** This powerful herb ties with CB2 receptors liable for directing irritation and torment. In view of its capacity to start a physiological reaction inside the ECS, its frequently used to treat osteoporosis and joint pain; and may possibly expand the adequacy of some enemy of malignant growth drugs.

- **Clove oil:** A strong segment of clove oil is eugenol – a ground-breaking cell reinforcement, mitigating, antimicrobial, and energizer. Beta-caryophyllene in cloves is a huge phytocannabinoid that can tie with CB2 receptors to diminish torment and irritation.

- **Echinacea:** You may be progressively familiar with echinacea as a virus cure, but this groundbreaking herb can also actuate CB1 receptors. It contains a compound called N-alkyl amides that are essentially the same as the effect of THC on torment, resistant framework, and irritation.

- **Peony:** This local bloom of China is an incredible wellspring of cannabinoids. Otherwise called peonia root, it is known for its capacity to decrease irritation in gout and other joint ailments, just as quieting muscle fits.

Appropriate Alternatives for Rick Simpson Hemp Oil

You may have known about Rick Simpson hemp oil. an oil that is fundamental from cannabis blossoms, it truly is high in the cannabinoid tetrahydrocannabinol (THC) and, as per Rick Simpson and others that are numerous has treated their malignant growth.

Does it truly work? Episodic proof clearly tips for the explanation that way. Unfortuitously, because of the shame cannabis that is encompassing cannabis, barely any medical research reports have endeavored. This is surely quickly changing, anyway for the present, there's definitely no unmistakable arrangement.

The Story of Rick Simpson Hemp Oil

Rick Simpson is extremely A Canadian specialist who endured awful damage that offered him ringing that is consistent with the ears. The ailment genuinely influenced their disposition, their ability to center, alongside his life. None with respect to the medicine specialists recommended worked. an episode of "The Nature of Things" that talked concerning the potential that is medical of incited Rick Simpson to concentrate oil through the plant to use to manage their disease. In spite of the fact that the ringing was by and by here, the oil previously got it down intensely to a useful degree. He had been in a situation to rest by and by, his inconvenience wound up being under wraps, and along these lines had been their pulse levels. Rick Simpson recovered his life right.

A few years after the fact, Rick found three spots on their skin which were analyzed as epidermis malignant growth tumors. One spot had been precisely disposed of, together with the other two had been to be killed some time. As Rick Simpson recovered, he reviewed a 1974 news report that referenced the aftereffects of THC on malignant growth tumors cells in mice. He endeavored the oil on his two staying spots, and multiple times they surely were gone. When the malignant growth that was killed returned two or after three weeks, he oversaw it as a result of the oil, and again his skin had been recuperated.

Rick Simpson wanted the entire globe to get some answers concerning their finding and began offering his oil for nothing out of pocket to malignant growth tumors exploited people. Various were recuperated. Unfortuitously, numerous specialists when you take a gander at the medical field responded contrarily to Rick Simpson's story. at long last ready to give their story to a more extensive group of spectators at whatever point movie producer Christian Laurette made a narrative "Go Through the Cure" about Rick Simpson's life finding. The narrative incited research by Spanish researchers on people groups disease tumors patients that broke down the consequences of THC on malignancy tumors cells. found that THC had assaulted the malignant growth tumors cells while making the tissue that is healthy it unblemished. In any case, Rick Simpson hemp oil keeps on being perhaps not proper spots, not just since it contains THC since it is gotten from cannabis, at the same time, the psychoactive fixing in the plant. Another elective that is legal cannabidiol.

CANNABIDIOL AND CANCER

Cannabidiol (CBD) could be the other cannabinoid that is major in cannabis blooms. In contrast to THC, CBD simply isn't psychoactive and it is getting used to managing youthful ones with obstinate epilepsy. CBD additionally experiences lower levels of medical research, however basically like research encompassing THC, the measure of studies is expanding, and introductory discoveries are ensuring. We at present comprehend that CBD can slow the advancement of and limit its forcefulness, it might truly be more advantageous than THC. Like its psychoactive cousin, CBD had been found to keep healthy bosom tissue unblemished. Other research reports have found that CBD is successful against prostate disease tumors and lung malignancy.

Legal Sources of Cannabidiol

Not absolutely a wide range of cannabidiol fits in many states. CBD acquired from medical marijuana suitable in states where medical cannabis itself is legal. Regardless, it could be expelled from mechanical hemp, prompting oil that contains for all intents and purposes no THC. This oil is "hemp is approved to be utilized being a nourishment added substance by the FDA into the United states and can be gotten legally and used countrywide.

As indicated by the INCB, the licit utilization of cannabis has expanded significantly since 2000. From that point forward, an ever-increasing number of nations have begun to utilize cannabis and additionally cannabis extricates for medical purposes, notwithstanding logical research. In 2000, all out production was 1.3 tons; by 2015, it had expanded to 100.2 tons. Revealed necessities for 2017 demonstrate further development to almost 160 tons. The current encounters of setting up approaches empowering access to therapeutic cannabis are shifted and the various procedures that prompted these strategies can for the most part be arranged as pursues:

- Individual cases safeguarded in the courts which set points of reference, or sentences that are applied for the most part, similar to the case in Mexico and Canada

- Direct just procedures, for example, referenda and prominent discussions like in a few US states

- Legislative and open approach procedures drove by national or sub-national governments, as in Uruguay and different US states

- Companies were creating therapeutic cannabis and requesting that administration specialists encourage their licit use, for instance in the UK.

Logical Audit of Cannabis by The United Nations

Aside from the basic leadership process, different elements can impact the sort and effect of the different administrative encounters. These incorporate the sort of society wherein the cannabis discussion happens, the level of improvement of its instructive and scholastic foundations, the quantity of experts devoted to considering the issue, the presence of a composed common society, the verifiable and social association with the plant, regardless of whether there are zones where cannabis is as of now being delivered in a nation, interest for cannabis and its subordinates for restorative or remedial purposes, and the open approach objectives sought after.

This can clarify the wide scope of reactions from nations to the interest for restorative cannabis use, which might be monetarily liberal like in the United States, or significantly statist on account of Uruguay (where open foundations handle all exercises identified with the production, preparing and closeout of cannabis). The encounters likewise vary with respect to characterizing restorative use, the sorts of products considered as medicines (for instance, a few nations just approve pharmaceuticals, for example, Sativex, while others permit home grew or non-pharmacological arrangements), regardless of whether development for individual use or the utilization of salves and oils is allowed, and so on. It is additionally important here that, even in instances of therapeutic guidelines, different types of cannabis use stay denied, with its hallowed utilize just permitted in Jamaica and recreational utilize just allowed in Uruguay and some US states. At last, different nations are at the underlying phase of the exchange, with proposed enactment viable in Costa Rica, Cyprus, Lithuania, Luxemburg, New Zealand, Saint Vincent and the Grenadines and South Africa.

Latin America And the Caribbean: New Pioneers in Therapeutic Cannabis Change

Latin America is at present the world chief in the advancement and appropriation of strategies enabling access to cannabis for helpful employments. Uruguay is the main nation on the planet to totally legalize the cannabis advertises for medical and logical purposes, just as for modern and recreational use. In this little nation, the state with help from the Institute for the Regulation and Control of Cannabis figures out who can create cannabis, just as how much and who can devour it, under which conditions. From one perspective, the administrative system for recreational use depends on giving licenses to people keen on planting, developing, collecting, delivering and commercializing cannabis, and incorporates a few types of access: self-development for individual use, cannabis clubs or buy in drug stores. These are totally unrelated, and the measure of cannabis that can be gained is constrained to 40g a month. On the other hand, the administrative framework for helpful cannabis sadly keeps on confronting different difficulties, including the way that the Ministry of Public Health doesn't approve the residential closeout of therapeutic cannabis.

Thus, patients wishing to get to restorative cannabis can just secure it inside the framework made for recreational purposes (that is, by delivering it themselves or getting to/buying a product that has not experienced all the logical testing vital for a medicine). An individual requiring treatment with Sativex or Marinol must demand an 'orange remedy' (the most confined solution) and round out an application routed to the Ministry of Public Health to acquire the consent to import the product from abroad. In the event that the application is acknowledged, the expense of the product remains amazingly high. The Chilean case is unique, in spite of the fact that somehow or another like the Uruguayan experience. Despite the fact that there was no change of Law 20, 000 patients requiring restorative cannabis can get to it by means of medical solutions (Decree 84 of the Institute for Public Health). In unique conditions, cannabis-based drugs can be approved for import, applications must be sent to the health authority taking care of enlistments.

The administrative organization is called ANAMED (Agencia Nacional del Medicamiento). As the drug stays difficult to reach in drug stores, the medical remedy can be utilized as a legal avocation of restorative use in court, which is permitted under article 4 of Law 20,000. This empowers patients to develop plants at home (no predefined number) or to be an individual from an aggregate cannabis development club, inasmuch as the last is directed under Law 20,500 on non-benefit resident cooperation. What's more, an undertaking drove by the Daya Foundation, related to the University of Valparaiso, Farmacopea Chilena and Knop Laboratories, expects to build up a phyto pharmaceutical that would be financially available.

Different nations, for example, Colombia, have likewise gained some ground. Law 1787, affirmed in 2015, made an administrative system for medical and logical access to cannabis, inside which the state holds command over the market and awards licenses to private elements for production, make, fare, change and research.66 When setting up the new administrative structure, the administration contemplated the way that cannabis was at that point being developed by subsistence ranchers in certain locales of Colombia and the law solicitations authorized makers to purchase their crude material legitimately from these little cultivators. This is a significant move to join the requirements of existing little scale cannabis ranchers in the new arrangement system. Be that as it may, specialized help is required for little cultivators to have the option to create crops that meet the necessary criteria for therapeutic cannabis.

Medicines created are phyto pharmaceuticals and can be gotten in approved drug stores, without a medical solution. The administration will expect to set a value that ensures access for all. Colombia is at present the nation that has enlisted the most elevated restorative cannabis yield with the INCB for 2018.In Jamaica, cannabis for therapeutic or remedial purposes must be suggested or endorsed by an enrolled doctor or a health expert guaranteed by the Ministry of Health. The import of cannabis products by patients is permitted as long as the doctor guarantees that the patient is experiencing a disease. In any case, not many experts endorse cannabis as a medicine. Visitors or individuals who don't dwell in Jamaica can apply for a license that enables them to buy and have up to two ounces (56 grams) of ganja. To do as such, they should display a specialist's solution or sign a willful announcement expressing their medical condition. With the primary approvals dating from 2014, Brazil has since permitted the importation of prescriptions dependent on CBD oil, including THC and marijuana blossoms in 2016, for medical and restorative use.

In any case, the Brazilian Federal Medical Board disallows the medicine by specialists of marijuana in its vegetal structure, under extraordinary conditions. Import requires consistence with a progression of necessities set up by the National Health Surveillance Agency (Agencia Nacional de Vigilancia Sanitaria, ANVISA). These incorporate patients' enrollment, taking care of managerial systems for import face to face, and applying for a license from the office. The probability of self-development of cannabis for such purposes stays under exchange. Argentina, Peru and Mexico have additionally embraced other, less aspiring, administrative procedures. In those nations, changes came about because of dynamic weight from common society and patients' gatherings, prompting the endorsement of approaches considering the deal and utilization of therapeutic cannabis. In October 2017, Peru endorsed its 'Law directing the restorative and remedial utilization of cannabis and its subsidiaries', which was marked by President Pablo Kuczynski on sixteenth November.

The law presents the utilization of libraries for the different gatherings who wish to get to cannabis (for example patients, shippers, research elements and open substances), and an arrangement of government licenses for research, importation, commercialization and production. It is significant that the nation has perceived the advantages of cannabis for the treatment of indications brought about by infections, for example, disease or numerous cases of sclerosis. In any case, the administrative system that will guarantee legal access to the substance stays to be explained. In Argentina, then, a standard was given that enables patients to import their prescription while the state starts the nearby production of pharmaceuticals for the domestic market.

In Mexico, the changes to the General Health Law and the Criminal Code in 2017 presently permit the utilization of cannabis for medical and logical purposes. The Ministry of Health was requested to give an open arrangement on the issue to guarantee that patients approach pharmacological products with and without THC. At long last, Bolivia is the most recent Latin American nation to date to have revised its medication enactment to permit therapeutic cannabis. Concurred inside the casing work of a more extensive medication enactment embraced on sixteenth March2017, people and organizations must enlist and demand an earlier approval to the Ministry of Health for the import, fare, exchange or production of therapeutic cannabis. Extraordinary and restricted approvals may likewise be allowed by the Ministry of Health for research on restorative cannabis.

North America: Pioneer in The Medicinal Cannabis Industry

The United States and Canada might be the most exceptional nations in the advancement of a therapeutic cannabis industry. In the United States, 29 states directly have an authorization allowing remedial cannabis use, similarly as the advancement, production, getting ready, arrangement and assessment gathering of cannabis and its subordinates. The United States is in this way a genuine case of blended procedures in with blended outcomes where the two choices and administrative procedures reacted to various needs and interests, mirroring an intriguing mixture of administrative systems that sway between those organizing general health and those seeking after real business finishes and income producing objectives:

- 14 states have legalized restorative cannabis by choice: California in 1996; Washington, Oregon and Alaska in 1998; Maine in 1999; Nevada, Hawaii and Colorado in 2000; Montana in 2004; Michigan in 2008; Arizona in 2010; and North Dakota, Florida and Arkansas in 2016

- 15 states have taken the administrative course: Vermont in 2004; Rhode Island in 2006; New Mexico in 2007; New Jersey in 2010; Delaware in 2011; Massachusetts and Connecticut in 2012; New Hampshire and Illinois in 2013; Nueva York, Minnesota and Maryland in 2014; Pennsylvania and Ohio in 2016; and West Virginia in 2017.In Canada, there are around 44 authorized makers approved by the Ministry of Health, just as a large number of Canadians authorized to have and expend therapeutic cannabis. In the two cases, self-development is permitted insofar as it doesn't surpass six plants and use can be defended.

Europe: Positive However Constrained Advances

In Europe, close by entrenched models of therapeutic cannabis as in the Netherlands, the previous year has seen the appropriation of different restorative cannabis plans, specifically in Greece, Poland and Slovenia. Different nations have been increasingly mindful, concentrating solely on pilot ventures. The Netherlands, in the meantime, legalized the restorative utilization of cannabis in 2000, and made the Bureau for Medicinal Cannabis (BMC) making a solid pharmacological industry, driven by Bedrocan Medical Cannabis which has the imposing business model of all therapeutic cannabis production and conveyance. All cannabis going through the BMC is created by Bedrocan – which created and institutionalized residential interest and fare a portion of the five sorts of pharmaceutical cannabis flos (blossom) prescriptions arranged with various rates of THC and CBD. Therapeutic cannabis is delivered across the nation and constrained by the Medicinal Cannabis Agency. It tends to be acquired in drug stores for various pathologies, just when the patient is in control of a medical remedy.

Restorative use has expanded significantly over the previous decade, with more than 50,000 patients presently being recommended cannabis in the Netherlands. Germany has quite recently finished the authoritative changes important to grow the medical utilization of cannabis. Under the watchful eye of the new law that went in January 2017, patients could just access medical cannabis through a unique singular approval. Germany is currently one of the main nations on the planet to incorporate medical cannabis in the fundamental scope of meds that must be secured by both private safety net providers and open health services. A national Cannabis Agency was set up under the Federal Institute for Drugs and Medical Devices (BfArM) to supervise the new procedure, as recommended by the global medication settlements. The 2017 law likewise permits the improvement of residential production of cannabis, despite the fact that until further notice all cannabis meds proceed with imported, basically from the Netherlands.

Somewhere else in Europe, an absence of essential guidelines of therapeutic cannabis in nations like the United Kingdom and the Czech Republic has hampered access to these prescriptions for a huge number of patients. In the previous, the administration just allows the utilization of Sativex for patients with various cases of sclerosis, under medical remedy. The general health administration in the United Kingdom has additionally settled that each patient must compensation for their prescription, at the expense of about500 Euros a month. In the Czech Republic, despite the fact that the nation legalized medical cannabis in 2013, there is an atomic procedure for obtaining licenses to create, sell or buy products got from cannabis. There keeps on being vulnerability about the extension and capability of this change, both for the welfare of the patients and for the advancement of an industry that can add to the development in the accessible stockpile, which stays insufficient all through the mainland. As in the United Kingdom, the cost of the drug is additionally a significant test; since therapeutic cannabis isn't secured by the health protection framework. As expressed over, a few nations have as of late pushed forward with a change in the zone of therapeutic cannabis. In Poland, for instance, first November 2017 denoted the main day on which therapeutic cannabis could be sold in enrolled drug stores.

Patients need extraordinary consent from a local pharmaceutical investigator and a doctor certify by the Ministry of Health. The law just permits the importation of cannabis (essentially from the Netherlands), as opposed to household production or self-development. Likewise, in Slovenia, as of February 2018, the Decree on the order of unlawful drugs (Official Gazette of the Republic of Slovenia, no. 45/14, 22/16 and 14/17) enables medical specialists to recommend cannabinoid-based drugs (manufactured, characteristic and the alleged therapeutic cannabis), just as institutionalized buds and blossoming highest points of cannabis (despite the fact that the last stays to be completely executed by and by). This arrangement changes required moving cannabis from Group I to Group II in the rundown of illegal substances of Slovenia. The Ministry of Health is responsible for actualizing the therapeutic cannabis plot. On first March 2018 Greece received the bill 'Arrangements for the Production of final results of therapeutic cannabis'. It is vital that most of the parliamentary ideological groups bolstered the bill; in spite of the fact that resistance groups casted a ballot against the bill in the last vote.

The bill recommends that Greece's medical patients can get to therapeutic cannabis products, in acknowledgment of their advantages for explicit ailments. It additionally recommends that people can develop cannabis for the sole reason for delivering therapeutic cannabis products in the nation. At long last, the bill perceives the financial capability of therapeutic cannabis; with the making of new openings and the capability of sending out products to the universal market. At long last, in different nations, restorative cannabis is restricted to pilot ventures. In Denmark, for instance, cannabis for helpful designs is as yet illegal, however an experimental run program will start on first January 2018 for a predetermined number of patients with explicit health issues (for example various sclerosis, constant torment and sickness). Therapeutic cannabis additionally stays illegal in Ireland; however some pilot tasks are in progress, and a bill was passed by the Dail (Irish parliament) in December 2016, despite the fact that the law has not yet come into force.84Israel:

The Middle Eastern: Special Case

Today, there are more than 50 labs directing research on restorative cannabis in the different colleges and scholastic establishments of Israel. The thorough logical learning and investigation of chances for logical and modern advancement have driven Israel to attempt changes on cannabis that don't really coordinate with its methodology towards different drugs. The nation endorsed the therapeutic utilization of cannabis in 1992 and before long turned into an inside for logical research and improvement of cannabis assortments and mechanical products. The enactment is executed by an
146

uncommonly settled unit in the Ministry of Health, the Israeli Agency on Medical Cannabis (IMCA), which set up a controlling advisory group in a joint effort with the Israeli police, the Ministry of Agriculture and the Ministry of Economy, headed by one of the logical pioneers of the field: Prof Meshulam.

The IMCA issues a few sorts of licenses for development, extraction and bundling plants, and dispersion. The IMCA is additionally answerable for the approval of uncommon clinicians who are permitted to recommend cannabis to patients experiencing extreme torment and various different side effects. Extra diseases can be treated in emergency clinics as a major aspect of clinical preliminaries. By 2017, somewhere in the range of 40,000 patients were getting therapeutic cannabis.

Asia:

Despite the fact that Asia keeps on being at the front line of severe medication strategies, and restorative cannabis stays disallowed in Japan, Vietnam, Pakistan, Cambodia and Nepal. Be that as it may, there have been certain advancements in a few nations of the area. In India, the law recognizes two sorts of cannabis products: ganja (the blooming or fruiting highest points of the cannabis plant) and charash or hashish (cannabisresin), with regulations being increasingly loose for the previous. The nation as of now has some legal arrangements for the restorative and logical utilization of the plant, however these arrangements presently can't seem to be actualized. Since 2017, different political figures, including Maneka Ghandi and MP Dr. Dharamvir Ghandi, demonstrated their help to cannabis strategy change. In the region of research on therapeutic cannabis, the 2015 Phyto pharmaceutical Act was passed to quicken examinations on plant-based medicines, a move that has the capability of pulling in speculations into cannabis research from huge organizations.

In the Philippines, while President Duterte kept on pursuing his war on drugs the nation over, the House Committee on Health endorsed the Medical Compassionate Medical Cannabis Act in September 2016. The law forbids the utilization of cannabis in its crude structure, and stipulates that patients need earlier approval from a specialist, and the treatment will be conveyed in committed focuses with a unique permit from the Department of Health, in clinics. The Philippine Drug Enforcement Agency is answerable for the guideline and regulation of restorative cannabis, which can be utilized to treat different diseases, including joint inflammation, epilepsy and numerous sclerosis, among others. The bill additionally plans to make a research office on therapeutic cannabis. In the interim, in Thailand an open discussion was held in August 2016 to expel cannabis from Category 5 of the nation's medication enactment, and the Agricultural Council was entrusted with building up a proposition for the decriminalization of the substance for thought by the legislature. From first January 2017, hemp was decriminalized in 15 areas and six territories of the northern district.

Oceania:

Australia gaining ground: There have been huge advancements in Australia on the therapeutic cannabis front as of late. Since 2016 the nation has another national body that can issue licenses to cultivators and direct restorative cannabis crops with the goal that therapeutic marijuana can be developed in Australia. Medical specialists may supply a restorative cannabis product to a patient in the wake of advising the pertinent administrative power and acquiring earlier authorization

148

from the state or domain government division. This is done on a patient-by-tolerant premise and therapeutic cannabis can likewise be utilized for clinical preliminaries. Probably the most significant changes have happened at the state and region level. The territory of New South Wales originally induced wide-running therapeutic cannabis preliminaries and furnished the police with the power not to arraign critically ill patients utilizing cannabis for medical purposes.

Few kids with the most pessimistic scenario of medication inhabitant epilepsy can likewise be recommended restorative marijuana under a merciful access plot. Victoria was the principal state to set up a state-based therapeutic cannabis plan enabling youngster with serious epilepsy to be given the medication. The entirety of different states and domains have plans to empower access to therapeutic cannabis through remedy for organizing of conditions. Queensland built up the primary direction reports for health professionals in March 2017. In December 2017, the Commonwealth delivered the national rules for five conditions and distributed these on the Therapeutic Goods Administration site. New Zealand likewise presented the Misuse of Drugs Amendment Bill in December 2017 with the objective of making restorative cannabis accessible without criminal obligation.

Contemplations for Legislative Reform

Among the nation models introduced above, there is a wide scope of instruments accessible to guarantee access to therapeutic cannabis:

- Unique individual licenses to import and utilize restorative cannabis, while keeping up generally denials over the plant, however setting up special cases to the law to guarantee patients' entrance to cannabis (for example in Poland).

- Guideline of supply through the formation of a permitting framework conceded to people or private substances as indicated by the kind of movement they participate in (production, fabricate, send out, handling, research, transport or deal), inside which the state can assume different jobs – from focal control to negligible assertion through administrative bodies (for example in Colombia or Peru).

- Guideline of interest with systems enabling legal access to prescriptions or natural cannabis arrangements through: self-development, cannabis clubs, postal requests, deal in facilities or deal in drug stores (for example in Uruguay for recreational, and as a matter of course, therapeutic use).

- The plan and usage of open approaches that manage access to specific products, in consistence with the administrative framework set up for medicines (for example in Germany). Contingent upon the kind of administrative system and to what extent it has been set up, different effects have been recognized on the ground – notwithstanding the proof previously referenced above with respect to the health advantages of therapeutic cannabis:

- The fantasy around increments in illegal cannabis use as an immediate consequence of the usage of restorative cannabis administrative systems doesn't remain constant, particularly among youths for whom cannabis use commonness has stayed stable, in nations like the United States.

- Similarly, the quantity of auto collisions brought about by intense cannabis inebriation has not expanded perceptibly in purviews where the utilization of arrangements with THC or home-grown types of cannabis is allowed.

- There have been no recorded passing's brought about by cannabis; despite what might be expected, the endurance rate and personal satisfaction of patients have improved.

There has been no sharp ascent in wrongdoing, maybe there is even proof in some US states executing a therapeutic cannabis plot that the wrongdoing rates have dropped by as much as 13%.

RECOMMENDATIONS

The data accessible so far makes it conceivable to plot the accompanying arrangement recommendations:

- Legalize cannabis for restorative use, just as meds and helpful substances got from cannabis, for all afflictions distinguished by logical research, and not exclusively constraining access for a couple of self-assertively decided diseases.

- Immediately incorporate drugs got from cannabis in the essential scope of medicines, that is, without the requirement for legal activities requiring the state to do as such, and keeping away from additionally the significant expenses that individual importation of such prescription would include for every particular case.

- Reform the essential laws to make and distribute a spending plan to guarantee the steady age of logical research.

- Coordinate every single pertinent organization to streamline the different specialized and clean procedures that enable new drugs to arrive at the market rapidly, while continually guaranteeing the most noteworthy potential models for purchaser health security.

- Establish the components important to keep away from the making of imposing business models or a limitation of the market to a couple of explicit gatherings who might hold all licenses and deal licenses to the inconvenience of the health and financial welfare of the overall public.

- Include the patients in basic leadership procedures identified with the improvement of general enactment and regulations, in order to set up standards that react to their needs with regards to every particular state.

- Avoid building up self-assertive ideas (for instance, the centralization of a specific psychoactive substance) that would influence access or result in the denial of a medicine that contains those substances.

- Offer specialized help to doctors, giving them the instruments, they have to comprehend both the advantages and the health dangers of therapeutic cannabis.

- Implement government funded training and mindfulness raising efforts for the overall population and patients on restorative cannabis.

- Every authoritative measure ought to incorporate residential regulations for production, instead of being restricted to the importation of products. The subsequent administrative systems ought to likewise consider all estimates important to advance the incorporation of existing little scale producers and, to the extent that conceivable, do as such under conditions equivalent or progressively ideal to those conceded to new allow holders and additionally capital-serious remote industry.

- Small-scale ranchers associated with cannabis development for subsistence purposes ought to be engaged with the basic leadership procedures to empower the joining of their needs, and ought to get specialized help so they can take an interest in the 'matter' of therapeutic cannabis.

CONCLUSION

The way that Cannabis Pharmacy oil is free from the psychoactive THC compound, is the thing that, makes the products so engaging. For quite a long time, marijuana has been thought to give individuals health benefits. Be that as it may, the issue was that it was incomprehensible or testing to confine the psychoactive THC fixing from the health-giving cannabinoids. Cannabis Pharmacy oil is a superb, ease, low-reaction path for individuals to discover alleviation from certain health conditions without the mind-changing impacts of THC, or standard pharmaceutical drugs, which can accompany a large group of unfavorable, troubling symptoms. It is an all-common product, where the cannabinoids are separated from the hemp plant. The cannabinoids are then weakened with transporter oil, the most well-known being coconut oil or hemp seed oil. CBD oil represents cannabidiol, and it is a characteristic, expanding prevalent product utilized for treating a large group of illnesses, throbs, and agonies Cannabis Pharmacy oil comes in two primary sorts.

The principal type is made out of confined cannabinoids, while the subsequent kind is "wide range" CBD oil that envelops different parts present in the marijuana plant. The marijuana plant Cannabis Sativa has in excess of 100 substance mixes known as cannabinoids. These cannabinoids are what give CBD oil its capacity to mend and ease torment and other basic health issues. It's imperative to comprehend that the dynamic cannabinoids in CBD oil are not equivalent to THC or tetrahydrocannabinol. THC is the compound in the marijuana plant that makes an individual vibe "high." CBD, nonetheless, isn't psychoactive and can't make somebody high and is gotten from the governmentally

154

authorized modern hemp plant. All in all, the advantages of CBD oil are utilized to treat a scope of constant illnesses, most quiet ceaseless agony, joint pain, and nervousness. The advantages of CBD oil are not successful in treating intense diseases, or extreme health issues.

Do Not Go Yet; One Last Thing to Do

If you enjoyed this book or found it useful, I would be very grateful if you would post a short review on Amazon. Your support really does make a difference, and I personally read all the reviews so that I can get your feedback and make this book even better.

Thanks again for your support!

www.ingramcontent.com/pod-product-compliance
Lightning Source LLC
Chambersburg PA
CBHW070549220526
45467CB00003B/1140